CARDIAC EMERGENCIES

Aphorism I. Hippocrates
From Facade facing Quadrangle, Harvard Medical School, Boston

CARDIAC EMERGENCIES

AND RELATED DISORDERS

THEIR MECHANISM, RECOGNITION

AND MANAGEMENT

By HAROLD D. LEVINE, M.D.

Senior Associate in Medicine, Peter Bent Brigham Hospital, Boston, Mass.
Assistant Clinical Professor of Medicine, Harvard Medical School

▶

LANDSBERGER MEDICAL BOOKS, INC.

New York

PREFACE

While practicing in rural New Hampshire I was called
on the telephone to attend a woodsman who had been
unable to reduce his hernia. It happened that I had not previously had occasion to reduce a strangulated hernia. Before
leaving my office I therefore thumbed hurriedly through John
Homans' "Textbook of Surgery" and, to my delight, found there
precise directions for "performing taxis," quoted directly from
Sir Astley Cooper. Having thus familiarized myself with the
procedure I had no difficulty whatever in reducing the patient's
hernia. I have had no occasion to repeat the technique since
that time. How this bit of useful information tucked away in
just the right place might sometime be of value to physician
and patient made a most profound impression upon me. If, as
seems current practice, an apology is necessary for the publication of a volume on a subject which has already been treated
elsewhere, perhaps this experience may be offered in expiation
—and the hope that some of the material presented here may
prove to be of similar value to others.

This monograph is the outgrowth of a series of seminars
presented during the last fifteen years to fourth-year students
of the Harvard Medical School during their affiliation on the
Medical Service of the Peter Bent Brigham Hospital. This
monograph represents, I believe, a synthesis of the "main-
stream" of medical thinking at the Peter Bent Brigham Hospital, of my own experience and of what reading I have managed
to do. It is inevitable that the written and spoken word of
each of my colleagues and the consensus of conferences with
students, House Officers, Assistant Residents and Residents
should leave their mark here. In preparing the text I soon found,
if I did not already realize, that familiarity with all of the literature on this subject of emergencies is quite impossible. The

[5]

most that can be aspired is an acquaintance with the more important sources. Each contribution read brings to light in geometrical progression a growing avalanche of additional references. As a practicing physician it would have been impossible for me to read them all.

It is inevitable that there will be considerable difference in the preparation and experience of the readers. An attempt has been made so to formulate the text that it may prove of interest and value to such a diverse group as cardiologists, internists, general practitioners of medicine and students. It is intended neither as an introduction to the subject nor as a summary of recent advances in the field. Emphasis has varied. In some portions I have gone into rather minute detail in procedures; in others, where this has not seemed necessary, I have sketched in a bare outline. For the most part I have tried to hew closely to the line of the immediate emergency and have tried to avoid the tendency to metamorphosis from monograph to textbook. On the other hand, especially where long-run thinking enters into the handling of the acute emergency—as it frequently does—or where long-term therapy is itself subject to acute catastrophe, these considerations have been discussed. An attempt is made not only to outline or detail plans of management, but, to the best of our knowledge, to explain the mechanism of the syndromes being considered and the mode of action of therapy. Though this is perhaps not a wholly necessary objective, this may be satisfying to those who like to consider themselves rational.

The following members of the Senior Staff were good enough to read over and criticise those portions of the earlier versions of the manuscript whose subject matter fell within the particular sphere of their own interest: Drs. Lewis Dexter, Dale G. Friend, Frank H. Gardner, Richard Gorlin, Roger B. Hickler, Samuel A. Levine, Bernard Lown and H. Richard Tyler of the Medical Service, and Drs. Harrison Black, Chilton Crane,

PREFACE

Edward A. Edwards, J. Hartwell Harrison, Francis D. Moore and Leroy D. Vandam of the Surgical Service. Dr. Eli Friedman made some of the photographic illustrations. To each and everyone I express my sincerest appreciation. Dr. Eugene C. Eppinger deserves a special tribute for reviewing the entire manuscript. It is a pleasure also to acknowledge my gratitude to my chief, Dr. George W. Thorn, for his advice and counsel. To W. B. Saunders Company I am indebted for permission to reproduce Figures 8 and 27A of this treatise from Dr. Samuel A. Levine's Clinical Heart Disease and the present Figure 23 from Levine and Harvey's Clinical Auscultation of the Heart, to Landsberger Medical Books, Inc. for permission to reproduce Figure 21 from Lown and Levine's Atrial Arrhythmias, Digitalis and Potassium, to Dr. Dwight E. Harken for Figure 35, to Warner-Chilcott Laboratories for permission to copy Figure 5, to Mrs. Wilhelmina Baert for her diligent copyreading and to Mrs. Ethel P. Wiggin for her invaluable assistance in typing the revisions of the script and in correcting the syntax. I am most grateful also to Mrs. Katherine Metcalf Allen for continued help and cooperation. And, last but not least, may I here express my most apologetic thanks to my wife, Barbara, and to my sons, Jeffrey and Jonathan, for their patience and fortitude during the long period of neglect and preoccupation incidental to the completion of this work.

Dedicated to My Teachers

HENRY A. CHRISTIAN

MONROE J. SCHLESINGER

SAMUEL A. LEVINE

CONTENTS

CHAPTER ONE

ACUTE LEFT VENTRICULAR FAILURE   21

"Bloodless Phlebotomy"
Phlebotomy
Oxygen Therapy
Digitalis
Hypotensive Measures

CHAPTER TWO

CARDIOGENIC SHOCK AND THE HYPOTENSIVE STATE   39

Pressor Amines
Digitalis

CHAPTER THREE

CARDIOGENIC CHEST PAIN — THE CORONARY EMERGENCIES   53

Angina Pectoris
Coronary Insufficiency
Acute Myocardial Infarction
Intravenous Therapy in Coronary Artery Disease
"Arm Chair" Treatment
Anticoagulant Therapy

[9]

CONTENTS

CHAPTER FOUR

UNUSUAL AND NON-CARDIAC CAUSES OF CHEST PAIN   87

Dissecting Aneurysm of the Aorta
Acute Mediastinal Emphysema
Nerve Root Pain
Rupture of the Esophagus
Acute Pericarditis
Chest Wall Pain
  Anterior Chest Wall Syndrome
  "Precordial Catch"
Hiatus Hernia and Peptic Esophagitis
Spontaneous Pneumothorax

CHAPTER FIVE

PULMONARY EMBOLISM, PULMONARY INFARCTION AND ACUTE COR PULMONALE   115

Clinical Syndrome
Physical Examination
Laboratory Findings
Importance of Leg Vein Thrombosis
Treatment—General Measures
Anticoagulant Therapy
Vein Ligation

CHAPTER SIX

"REFRACTORY" CONGESTIVE HEART FAILURE   133

Review of Diagnosis
Review of Treatment

CONTENTS

Use of Mechanical Measures
Malabsorption of Digitalis
Electrolyte Imbalance
Low Sodium Syndrome
Tandem Diuretic Therapy. Steroid Therapy
Optimism in Therapy

CHAPTER SEVEN

OTHER ELECTROLYTE DISTURBANCES AS CARDIO-VASCULAR EMERGENCIES   155

Potassium Intoxication
Potassium Depletion

CHAPTER EIGHT

DIGITALIS INTOXICATION   173

Subjective Manifestations
Arrhythmias
Treatment

CHAPTER NINE

PAROXYSMAL ATRIAL TACHYCARDIA   191

Diagnosis
Differential Diagnosis
Treatment

CHAPTER TEN

ATRIAL FLUTTER   215

Differential Diagnosis
Treatment

[11]

CONTENTS

CHAPTER ELEVEN

ATRIAL TACHYCARDIA WITH BLOCK   235

Electrocardiographic Features
Differential Diagnosis
Management

CHAPTER TWELVE

ATRIAL FIBRILLATION   249

Diagnosis
Differential Diagnosis
Management
Special Considerations

CHAPTER THIRTEEN

PAROXYSMAL VENTRICULAR TACHYCARDIA   263

Electrocardiographic Diagnosis
Differential Diagnosis
Alternating Bidisectional Ventricular Tachycardia
Treatment

CHAPTER FOURTEEN

ADAMS-STOKES DISEASE   291

Diagnosis
Management
Ventricular Tachysystole in Complete Heart Block

CONTENTS

CHAPTER FIFTEEN

SYNCOPE 313

Vaso-Depressor Syncope
Syncope due to Impaired Venous Return
Cardiac Syncope
Cerebral Syncope

CHAPTER SIXTEEN

CARDIAC ARREST AND RESUSCITATION 333

The Anticipated or Imminent Emergency
Recognition of Cardiac Arrest
Management of Ventricular Standstill
Procedure for Ventricular Fibrillation

CHAPTER SEVENTEEN

MISCELLANEOUS EMERGENCIES 353

Pericardial Tamponade
Venous Air Embolism
Fat Embolism

INDEX 365

INTRODUCTION

A PHILOSOPHY FOR

EMERGENCIES

Ordinarily we think of an emergency as an unforeseen, abruptly developing predicament which jeopardizes life or limb and which demands immediate action if the patient or member is to survive. In this restricted sense emergencies are not common in clinical practice. Though in rare instances an emergency may present itself for "instant" solution, it is more commonly present continuously over a limited period of time. But this serious situation cannot last indefinitely. The concept of an emergency may be further broadened to include even states which are insidious in onset and in which there may be considerable latitude in time for a careful consideration of a course of therapy. In this expanded sense emergencies are not uncommon. An unrecognized, but potentially reversible, subacute or chronic condition may threaten the survival of the individual just as emphatically as such a well-recognized acute emergency as acute left ventricular failure. In subacute bacterial endocarditis, for example, there must be some point in time before which the condition is, and beyond which it is not, totally or partially reversible. The emergency here may relate simply to the question whether or not the attending physician will consider this possibility in time. To treat this type of emergency would require a large-scale incursion into the entire field of internal medicine. Most of the cardiac emergencies fall somewhere between these extremes. The emergency characteristically develops catastrophically but ample time is available for deliberation, reading or even consultation. It is implicit in this concept that there must be something that can be and should be done favorably to alter this situation.

Beginning in our medical school days all of us have developed frames of thought for dealing with emergencies. It is, I suspect, a favorite exercise of the physician en route to a stricken patient to review the various possible reasons why he has been called. From the gist of the telephone message the physician will in his own mind have reviewed the more prominent diagnostic possibilities before he arrives on the scene and will have thought out the therapeutic procedures appropriate to each situation even to the order in which they might be applied. The present treatise represents in part a compilation of this type of thinking regarding the cardiac emergencies encountered in clinical practice. It aims to establish first a general strategy with reference to each of these situations and then to outline, in some detail, the tactics which might then be employed. It is recognized that sagacity plays an important rôle at the critical moment. But by and large important decisions are not made in haste; appropriate emergency action springs rather from the prepared posture of sound emergency thinking already accomplished.

The summoned physician just described cannot help but reflect that what appears to a layman or even to another physician as a potentially disastrous situation may not at all impress him as such. Every contingency must be considered from this point of view. Is this really an emergency or does it merely seem to be? What appears to be but is not a true emergency demands not prompt action, but prompt reassurance and inaction.

Very few of the therapeutic measures to be detailed here have been subjected to the test of critical scientific evaluation. It is difficult if not impossible to carry out entirely satisfying scientific research on management. To illustrate, it seems ironical that the conclusions derived from one large scale attempt to study the efficacy of a form of therapy, namely that of anticoagulants in acute myocardial infarction, using the alternate case technique, should have become the subject of so much disagreement. If physicians cannot agree on the conclusions derived from a deliberate and extensive study of this sort, how can they be expected to agree on the value of the many other drugs and procedures which have been the subject of cruder, sparser and less painstaking observation?

Some of these practices may be founded more upon faith or hope than science and many will in time be proven to be ill-founded. Despite the onslaught of the gadgeteers there is still much that is empirical in medicine. The use of tourniquets in acute pulmonary edema, for example, is based upon the premise that their application traps blood in the extremities and reduces the "effective" blood volume. But it has been demonstrated recently that such an effect is probably negligible.[1] Yet there is very little doubt of the effectiveness of this treatment. At any rate these emergencies will continue in the foreseeable future to require our attention. And, in the last analysis, even if it's for the wrong reason, a particular form of therapy should be used, and continue to be used, so long as it works, or seems to work, until another is proven to be more effective. This brings to mind a gentle rebuke by Dr. Henry Christian. In presenting a patient to him on weekly rounds, a house physician, well aware of Dr. Christian's reputation as a therapeutic nihilist, made a particular point of being utterly objective about the efficacy of the patient's treatment. In summing up he stated that the patient had done well after he had received a certain preparation but that he was not certain that this improvement was the result of the particular medication used. "Yes," was Dr. Christian's reply, "but we like to believe that it was!"

The emergency may have a very important dividend. In the excitement and hurry of the acute emergency the physician is prone to rush through his procedure, by-passing unessentials and omitting the recording of data. This is understandable and frequently unavoidable. But the physician must bear in mind also that the acute emergency may well present a golden opportunity to make a definitive diagnosis which has not previously been possible. This is particularly true of syncopal attacks and arrhythmias. The examination, though hurried, should include certain critical information. One of the purposes of this presentation is to indicate what these data might be. And these findings should be recorded just as soon as possible after emergency therapy has been given.

A word about the "emergency physician," that post-war newcomer to the American scene who has been so designated by the public. The proper management of these emergencies may be a troublesome chore, it may be time-consuming and inconvenient and it may be technically demanding. Frequently this duty falls to the lot of a physician who is not the patient's regular medical attendant. It may devolve on the "emergency physician" who is called through the telephone service. In some communities this means the profession at large taking its turn in this important responsibility. In others it has become synonymous with the younger, unestablished members of the profession. To the latter this has offered an unsurpassed opportunity to set up the beginning of a successful practice. To all it represents an excellent contact with one of the most challenging and satisfying aspects of the practice of medicine.

REFERENCE

(1) Samet, P., Bernstein, W. H. and Boucek, R. J.: Effect of rotating tourniquets upon plasma volume and red cell mass. Proc. 32nd Scientific Sessions, Am. Ht. Ass'n., Oct. 23-24, 1959. p. 763.

1

ACUTE LEFT VENTRICULAR FAILURE

"Bloodless Phlebotomy"

Phlebotomy

Oxygen Therapy

Digitalis

Hypotensive Measures

1

ACUTE LEFT VENTRICULAR

FAILURE

This is one of the most frequent, most dramatic and most
serious of all medical emergencies. It is generally quite
easily recognized. Characteristically the patient is wakened from
a sound sleep in the early hours of morning, struggling franti-
cally against a feeling of overwhelming suffocation and ter-
rorized by a fear of impending death. Particularly in patients
with mitral stenosis attacks may also occur during the day,
following unusual exertion.[1] The bubbling respirations are often
audible across a large room. At times the dyspnea may be
wheezing in type and the respiration quite like that characteristic of bronchial asthma. The patient breaks out in a sweat and
sits instinctively at the edge of his bed or on a chair or rushes
to an open window for more air. He frequently raises frothy and
sometimes pinkish sputum. Moist medium to loud bubbling
râles are heard throughout the lung fields or only at the lung
bases. They are often so loud as to make auscultation of the
heart extremely difficult if not impossible. After minutes or hours
the attack gradually subsides and the patient soon falls back
to sleep. The whole terrifying ordeal may repeat itself once
or more often during the remainder of the night. Occasionally
an attack ends fatally. The disorder occurs in patients with

hypertensive heart disease, aortic stenosis or regurgitation, mitral stenosis or in well established coronary artery disease. It may also develop for the first time during, or even be the presenting clinical feature of, an acute attack of myocardial infarction.

Generally diagnosis presents no real problem. At times, however, bronchospasm makes confusion possible with chronic pulmonary disease in general and bronchial asthma in particular. The finding of clubbed fingers or a pronounced degree of cyanosis, a history of allergic diseases, persistence of wheezing between attacks or the demonstration of pulmonary parenchymal lesions or of right ventricular enlargement by roentgenray, electrocardiogram or physical examination, point in favor of chronic pulmonary disease. Bronchial asthma may generally be differentiated from cardiac asthma by the absence of moist râles during an attack or of severe dyspnea between attacks, by the small size of the heart in patients affected with this disease and by the scanty and mucoid rather than abundant, frothy and pinkish sputum. In some cases, particularly those not previously known to the physician, a differentiation between bronchial asthma and pulmonary congestion due to heart disease cannot be made.

In many cases simple measures are rapidly effective in aborting an attack; in others recourse must be had to a series of procedures or drugs of increasing complexity. If the patient is not already in a sitting position of his own accord, he should be seated upright in a chair and given a hypodermic injection of 10 to 15 mgms. of morphine. This is preferred to the more rapidly acting intravenous route (4–8 mgms.); generally a hypodermic is quite speedily effective. Since morphine may not be absorbed from a subcutaneous site in severe shock the intravenous route would then be preferred. If the patient vomits as a result of this injection, as he frequently does, he may be given 5 mgms. of prochlorperazine (Compazine) intramuscularly;

such an experience would indicate the substitution of Demerol (50–75 mgms.) in a subsequent paroxysm. Morphine is one of the most useful drugs in the treatment of pulmonary edema. Why a respiratory depressant should be so effective is not clear. It may be related to its effect in allaying anxiety or to the depression of respiratory labor and to the resulting decrease in venous return and in cardiac work.[2] By way of digression it must be emphasized that morphine is dangerous in bronchial asthma and in the congestive heart failure associated with severe chest deformities ("pulmono-cardiac failure"). It should not be used in these conditions even in minimal doses.

"BLOODLESS PHLEBOTOMY"

If pulmonary edema persists, venous tourniquets should be applied. The physician would be well-advised to carry four 1½ foot lengths of stout, narrow bore, ¼″ outer diameter, ⅛″ caliber diameter (Bittner Brand #876) rubber tubing in his bag. These are applied about the upper arms and thighs as close to the axillae and groins as is comfortable. They should be bound with a slip-knot, as in performing an ordinary venesection, at a pressure somewhere between the systolic and diastolic levels; that is, tight enough to prevent venous return but not so tight as to interfere with arterial flow into the limb. For observation of the blood pressure during the procedure a sphygmomanometer cuff may be used as the fourth tourniquet. I know of no good reason why, at the outset, one need be restricted to the use of three rather than four tourniquets. These trap or pool a considerable volume of blood in the extremities and proportionately decrease the venous return to the heart. This simple expedient is frequently adequate to relieve the overburdened heart and thus to permit the patient to recover from his attack. The patient generally recognizes his impending improvement long before objective evidence for this is actually at hand. In fact râles may

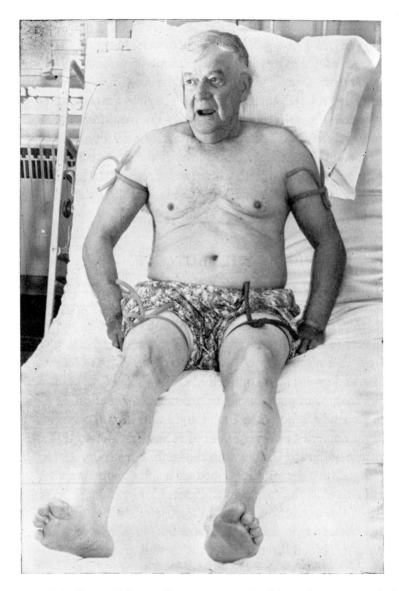

Fig. 1. *"Bloodless Phlebotomy."* Tourniquets of rubber tubing are applied snugly about the four extremities as near the trunk as feasible. The constriction must not be so tight as to obliterate arterial pulsations.

persist at the bases or along the vertebral margins of the scapulae for hours after the attack. When improvement is obvious
the tourniquets may be released. To prevent sudden overwhelming of the heart with trapped blood, first, one tourniquet should
slowly and gently be loosened and removed. Then after a few
minutes, during which the effect of this tentative elimination is
assessed, a second tourniquet is similarly removed, and so on
until all are off. If the symptoms persist despite the application
of tourniquets, or return on their removal, it may be advisable
to keep them on for a prolonged period. It will then be necessary to relieve each of the extremities in turn of the discomfort
of constant venous occlusion. The tourniquet is removed in the
manner just described, first from, say, the right arm and kept
off for five minutes or so. It is then re-applied and the right leg
tourniquet similarly removed, then re-applied, then the left leg,
then the left arm. Though proof is lacking, it seems reasonable
that, even if the use of tourniquets does not actually stop an
attack, it still must have a beneficial effect by sparing the heart
the extra load of the blood pooled in the extremities. This process
of "rotation of tourniquets" is frequently practiced for hours.
If the patient has many attacks of nocturnal dyspnea, as is
commonly the case, it is prudent to have rubber tubing of the
appropriate size on hand in the patient's room. The nurse or
some member of the family should be familiar with the proper
manner of applying tourniquets. This can save many unnecessary night calls. A recently suggested refinement of the rotating
tourniquet technique [3] employs blood pressure cuffs on the extremities and a valve which permits inflation of any three of
these to an identical pressure from a small carbon dioxide tank.
This apparatus has the virtue of the blood pressure cuff in general, namely that of distributing the pressure widely and thus
preventing local injury.

PHLEBOTOMY

If this procedure has been ineffective and the patient has a normal or elevated hematocrit and an elevated blood pressure, phlebotomy should be done. Even if the use of tourniquets has been successful, one should now consider phlebotomy, but in general the tendency will be to let well enough alone, perform a hematocrit determination in the morning and, if this is high, say over 45%, to proceed with phlebotomy at that time. Ordinarily a favorable response may not be anticipated except in an individual who has an elevated blood pressure at the time. Anemia would constitute another contraindication to proceeding with phlebotomy.

It has been my observation that there are many physicians, and this includes specialists as well as general practitioners, who have not performed a phlebotomy since the completion of their internships. This is very easy to understand. The techniques in vogue at the time of their training were cumbersome and, frequently, ineffectual. For example, a procedure, used 25 years ago or so, involved the use of a vacuum bottle or of a bottle provided with a two-hole rubber stopper, one of which was connected through a non-collapsible rubber tube to the phlebotomy needle, and the other through another tube to a Potain or similar aspirator. The many joints and connections were very prone to clot or leak, making necessary an embarrassed abandonment of the procedure after a token phlebotomy.

Fortunately these procedures have been largely abandoned. There seems to be general agreement that rapid bleeding is much more effective than slow bleeding in relieving the struggling heart of acute left ventricular failure. This does not necessarily mean that the bleeding must be fast. A time-honored, practically foolproof and rapid technique consists of the simple use of a 100 cc. glass syringe. A 15 gauge donor's needle or

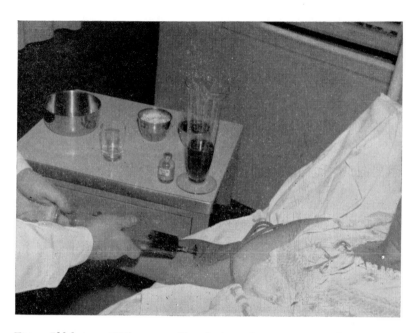

Fig. 2. *Phlebotomy With 100 cc. Glass Syringe.* Syringe is irrigated with citrate solution from tumbler before and between aspirations. Skin is prepared with iodine solution, then alcohol sponges; phlebotomy site is novocainized, tourniquet applied and phlebotomy needle, attached to 100 cc. syringe, introduced into vein. Four aspirations each of 125 cc. are successively and rapidly emptied into large beaker.

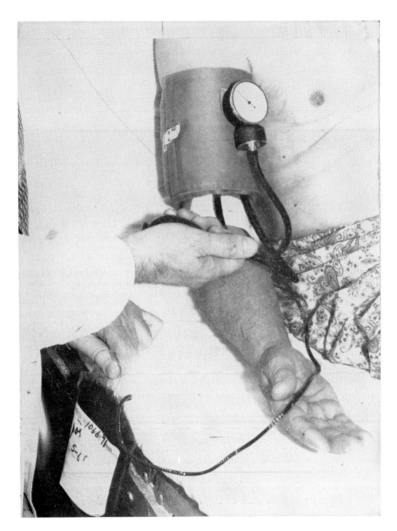

Fig. 3. *Phlebotomy With Plastic Bag.* One may apply tourniquet or blood pressure cuff inflated to pressure between systolic and diastolic levels. Skin is prepared as in Fig. 2, needle introduced into vein and blood allowed to siphon into collapsed dependent bag containing citrate solution. In patients with both shock and pulmonary edema, the tourniquet may be released, the bag elevated and turned upside down and the patient transfused with part of the removed blood in the event that he is overbled.

15 gauge short bevel intravenous needle is attached to the syringe which is first rinsed with citrate solution which has been placed in a tumbler and which is kept handy to the physician. One hundred twenty-five cc. of blood are rapidly drawn into the syringe, the syringe is rapidly emptied into a nearby milk bottle, the syringe again rinsed in citrate, re-attached, and the whole process repeated four times. Refinements of this technique are preliminary novocainization of the skin over the vein and the use of a short (2″) length of stout rubber tubing, provided with proximal and distal adapters and a clamp to prevent spilling between aspirations.

There are now available commercially a number of types of donor's sets consisting of needle, tubing and collapsed plastic bag containing citrate and into which the patient may be bled. Two or three may be carried in the doctor's bag. The bleeding consumes some 10 or 15 minutes but is generally quite effective. The removed blood may then stand the patient in good stead should he be overbled from pulmonary edema into shock. In that event he can be transfused with part of the blood which has just been removed. If the phlebotomy has been done in a hospital it may serve a double purpose, including the practical one of helping replenish the hospital blood bank. In transfusing patients who have recently been phlebotomized the preference will be to utilize packed red cells, not whole blood.

OXYGEN THERAPY

Since hypoxia is a common effect of pulmonary edema as well as an important contributory factor in its production,[4] oxygen will be given as early in the attack as feasible. Ordinarily preference will be given to the use of oxygen by nasal catheter. This is simpler and cheaper than other modes of administration. With a nasal catheter a level of 30% oxygen saturation can be attained in the upper respiratory passages, with tents

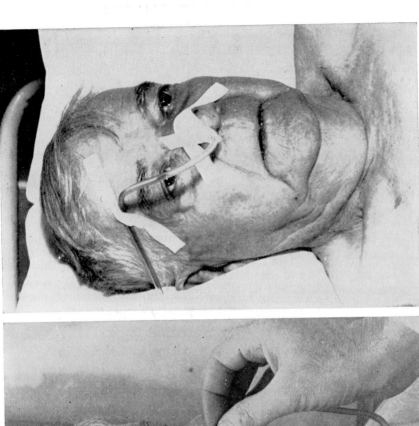

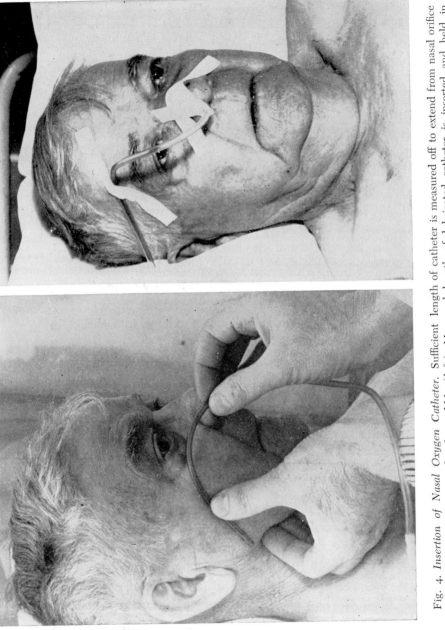

Fig. 4. *Insertion of Nasal Oxygen Catheter.* Sufficient length of catheter is measured off to extend from nasal orifice in curvilinear fashion to angle of mandible (left). Measured length of lubricated catheter is inserted and held in position by adhesive tape which binds catheter to nose and forehead (right). Proximal end of catheter is secured to sheet in back of head with a safety pin allowing enough length to permit mobility of head and neck.

60% and with various types of masks up to 100%. These techniques may be employed in those not responding to the nasal catheter, which is quite effective in most patients. It does tend to produce some local irritation of the nose and throat. The oxygen tent, on the other hand, is cumbersome to maintain and renders the patient relatively unavailable for other forms of therapy. The simple mask is all too apt to provoke panic on the part of the suffocating patient. For a time there was a vogue in the use of the positive pressure mask which has the theoretical advantages of decreasing the tendency to exudation of fluid from the pulmonary capillaries into the alveoli, of enabling the blood to carry more oxygen in simple physical solution [5] and of decreasing venous return to the heart. But it is very questionable if, as a practical matter, this technique actually accomplishes these purposes. It is worth remembering that in most communities the fire department or rescue squad is willing to provide emergency oxygen therapy. When they are to be summoned an unexcited person should deliver the message, make it clear that there is really not a fire, and that one or two men, tried and true, can handle the situation as well as, if not better than, an entire ladder company.

Oxygen should not be reserved for the use of those only with obvious cyanosis. Hypoxia may occur without cyanosis and cyanosis without hypoxia. Thus even if the patient is not cyanotic he may benefit from oxygen therapy. There is moreover considerable variation among us physicians in our ability to detect cyanosis.[6] We are frequently unable to detect cyanosis of like grade in different patients or in the same patient at different times. Few can interpret minor degrees of arterial oxygen unsaturation correctly. Some of us are even unable to recognize definite cyanosis when arterial oxygen saturation is as low as 71–75%.

It is ordinarily stated that a flow of 6 or 7 liters per minute should be maintained. This is empirical. Occasionally a flow up to 10 liters per minute will be necessary. It would be ideal to determine the patient's arterial oxygen saturation by femoral arterial puncture and repeat this determination after oxygen therapy has been started to see if oxygen flow is adequate, but this is obviously impossible in the heat of the emergency situation. One uses whatever form of oxygen therapy is available and is pleased if the patient obviously pinks up. There is no question that many patients with acute pulmonary edema feel much better during oxygen therapy, but, since the effect of oxygen must be slower than that of, say, tourniquets, it is very difficult to prove that it actually shortens or aborts attacks.

For patients who have frequent attacks of pulmonary edema an oxygen tank with all the necessary appurtenances should be available and in good running condition. The nurse or some-one in the family should be adept at its care and manipulation.

A new wrinkle in the use of oxygen is to bubble it through 95% alcohol instead of through water. This saturates the oxygen with alcohol vapor. By virtue of its effect in lowering surface tension, an "anti-foaming action" within the pulmonary alveoli, has been attributed to this technique. Clinical experience with this procedure has been encouraging [7,8]; the method awaits more extensive trial.

DIGITALIS

If the patient with acute pulmonary edema has received no digitalis within the previous two or three weeks he should be digitalized. This may be done orally over the course of two or three days if he has already improved, or intravenously with a rapidly acting digitalis preparation if therapy thus far has been ineffective. A technique for rapid oral digitalization is presented on page 226. For intravenous purposes one may use Digoxin 1.0 mgm., Cedilanid 0.8 to 1.2 mgms., Strophanthin K 0.3 mgm. or Strophanthin G (Ouabain) 0.5 mg. Since digitalis prevents recurrent attacks, it has seemed reasonable to regard the mere fact of acute pulmonary edema as warrant enough for continuous digitalis maintenance. Further details on intravenous digitalis administration are given on page 255.

In an occasional case one or two ampoules of aminophylline (0.24 to 0.48 gram) injected undiluted by vein over the course of a minute may afford striking relief of a paroxysm. This is the drug of choice where a differentiation between bronchial asthma and cardiac asthma has not been possible. Although it is felt by some workers that this medication is of value only if there is a prominent degree of bronchospasm, it has been our experience that it is frequently effective in acute pulmonary edema in general, even in the absence of bronchospasm. Although there is some apprehension about the too rapid injection of aminophylline, there is no convincing proof that this substance is more dangerous than any other substance given by vein. This will be discussed further under the subject of intravenous therapy in coronary artery disease (P. 65). It is well to warm the ampoule in a tumbler of warm water until it is at or about body temperature, a precaution which applies to all intravenous medication.

HYPOTENSIVE MEASURES

At times, particularly if given early in an attack, nitroglycerin 0.3 to 0.6 mgm. under the tongue will abort an attack. Just how this improvement comes about is uncertain. Some have attributed the improvement to the fall in blood pressure induced by the drug, some to the tourniquet-like effect of postarteriolar pooling of blood. Carotid sinus stimulation gently performed over seconds or minutes may be effective in producing a prompt and dramatic alleviation of the pulmonary signs and relief of dyspnea in patients with arterial hypertension.[9,10] But we cannot subscribe to the recommendation [10] that pressure over the carotid sinus may be continued for as long as half an hour.

In very resistant cases associated with hypertension ganglionic-blocking agents have been employed.[11] These agents should preferably be given under hospital control. Occasionally this has been successful where all other methods have failed. Arfonad has the virtue of titratable effects. The contents of a 5 cc. ampoule (50 mgms. are contained in 1 cc.) are dissolved in 250 cc. of 5% dextrose in water and infused at the rate of 10 drops (0.5 mgm.) per minute. The drip rate is gradually increased until a reduction of 25 to 30% in the blood pressure level is achieved. The pressure is maintained at this level until the patient is out of his attack. Intramuscular Serpasil may also be employed. (See page 326.)

On rare occasion acute hypertension and left ventricular failure may be the effect of peripheral embolism. Thus in mitral stenosis and atrial fibrillation with embolism it may be mandatory to attack the seeding source of embolism at the time of embolectomy. This problem will rarely arise except in relation to saddle aortic embolism; femoral emboli do not induce left ventricular failure and they can be removed under local anaesthesia in exceedingly "poor risk" patients. In severely ill mitral patients, on the other hand, the suddenly acquired hypertension which is associated with embolism to the aortic bifurcation or to both iliac arteries, may precipitate acute pulmonary edema. If hypertension persists aortic embolectomy should be done first. If, on the other hand, the blood pressure falls, the strategy should be first, relief of the tight mitral stenosis; then embolectomy.

Renal infarction may attain the status of an acute emergency when the patient has only one kidney. A 65 year old woman was recently admitted in a state of anuria of four days' duration with arterial hypertension and acute left ventricular failure. Ureteral catheterization proved that the kidney was excreting no urine at all. Angiography showed evidence of obstruction in the renal artery. Endarterectomy and partial nephrectomy resulted in resumption of function of this kidney and great improvement in her circulatory and renal status.[12]

At times acute pulmonary edema may be the sole or predominant manifestation of active myocardial infarction, of acute pulmonary embolism or of paroxysmal rapid heart action of any type. These may render ineffective any or all of the above-described measures. Failure of improvement should suggest one of these possibilities if previously unsuspected. Treatment must then be directed toward this background process.

REFERENCES

(1) Lombardo, T. A. and Harrison, T. R.: Cardiac asthma. Circulation 4: 920, 1951.

(2) Visscher, M. B., Haddy, F. J. and Stephens, G.: The physiology and pharmacology of lung edema. Pharmacological Reviews. 8: 389, 1956.

(3) Seligman, H.: New apparatus for treatment of pulmonary edema. J.A.M.A. 161: 721, 1956.

(4) Drinker, C. K.: Pulmonary Edema and Inflammation. Harvard University Press. 1945, p. 29.

(5) Comroe, J. H., Jr. and Dripps, R. D.: The Physiological Basis for Oxygen Therapy. Charles C. Thomas, Springfield Illinois, 1953, p. 9.

(6) Comroe, J. H., Jr. and Botelho, S.: The unreliability of cyanosis in the recognition of arterial anoxemia. Am. J. Med. Sci. 214: 1, 1947.

(7) Lusiada, A. A.: Therapy of paroxysmal pulmonary edema by antifoaming agents. Circulation 2: 872, 1950.

(8) Gootnich, A., Lipson, H. I. and Turbin, J.: Inhalation of ethyl alcohol for pulmonary edema. N.E.J. Med. 245: 842, 1951.

(9) Wasserman, S.: Zum Mechanismus des akuten kardialen Lungenödems: mit Berücksichtigung eines elektrokardiographierten und durch Karotissinusdruck beendeten Anfalls. Cardiologia 3: 402, 1939.

(10) Alzamora-Castro, V., Battilana, G., Garrido-Lecca, G., Rubio, C., Abugattas, R. and Bouroncle, J.: Acute left ventricular failure and carotid sinus stimulation. J.A.M.A. 157: 226, 1955.

(11) Sarnoff, S. J., Goodale, W. T. and Sarnoff, L. C.: Graded reduction of arterial pressure by means of a thiophanium derivative (Ro2–2222). Preliminary observations on its effect in acute pulmonary edema. Circulation 6: 63, 1952.

(12) Merrill, J. P., Harrison, J. H. and Crane, C.: Unpublished observations.

2

CARDIOGENIC SHOCK AND

THE HYPOTENSIVE STATE

Pressor Amines

Digitalis

2

CARDIOGENIC SHOCK AND

THE HYPOTENSIVE STATE

The shock complicating such medical catastrophes as
myocardial infarction, pulmonary embolism, infarction
of the bowel, congestive heart failure, hemorrhage, severe overwhelming infection or drug intoxication is manifested not only
by a profound fall in blood pressure but by certain compensatory or secondary clinical findings. This includes a rapid thready
pulse, a cold clammy skin, ashen pallor and mottled cyanosis,
dyspnea, thirst, air hunger and certain cerebral symptoms such
as restlessness, faintness, stupor or coma. Occurring in acute
coronary thrombosis shock is a grave complication, being associated with a mortality rate of 80 to 90%. The drop in blood
pressure is probably the effect of an abrupt decrease in left
ventricular output.[1,2] The cold clammy skin and ashen pallor
are manifestations of compensatory peripheral vasoconstriction.
There is reason to believe that the latter mechanism may at
times be partly or wholly lacking. Thus, while most authorities
insist that there must be changes in both categories, namely
hypotension plus one or more of the enumerated clinical findings to justify the designation of shock, others feel that, regardless of whether signs of vasoconstriction are present, the
simple finding of profound and persistent hypotension means

shock and demands immediate and appropriate therapy. The self-perpetuating nature of shock has been emphasized repeatedly in the literature. The "vicious cycle" of shock in acute myocardial infarction, for example, is perpetuated by the diminished irrigation of coronary arteries other than those which are thrombosed, as a consequence of the fall in blood pressure.[3] This can lead to complicating multiple segmental infarcts or to subendocardial ischemia or infarction.

The patient in shock should be given morphine if he is in pain. Unless he is in congestive heart failure he should be placed in the Trendelenburg shock position. If failure is present some sort of compromise must be worked out between the feet-up and the head-up position.

Efforts to overcome the shock of myocardial infarction by measures aimed primarily at a restoration of blood volume, e.g., blood or plasma transfusion or the use of plasma-expanders (Dextran) have been disappointing.[4,5] They have entailed the definite risk of precipitating or aggravating congestive heart failure in general and acute pulmonary edema in particular. Intra-arterial transfusion has been offered as a safe substitute for intravenous transfusion [6] because of its alleged effect of avoiding pulmonary flooding and increasing coronary flow as a result of its direct effect of elevating aortic pressure.[7] Its superiority has been confirmed neither in the laboratory nor at the bedside.

PRESSOR AMINES

Until recently physicians have been reluctant to employ vasopressor substances in the treatment of shock in myocardial infarction. It was feared that these substances would predispose to the development of dangerous cardiac arrhythmias. It was believed moreover that these patients were already maximally vasoconstricted and that further vasoconstriction could not be anticipated, or that, if it did develop, it would increase capillary hypoxia and aggravate shock.[8] In spite of these forebodings various pressor amines have been utilized, at first tentatively and cautiously, but more recently in a considerable body of experience. The effectiveness of various amines such as phenylephrine hydrochloride (Neosynephrine),[9] mephentermine (Wyamine),[10] methoxamine (Vasoxyl),[11] metaraminol (Aramine),[12] and more particularly, nor-epinephrine or L-arterenol (Levophed) [8,13,14] has been substantiated. The use of these substances has been followed not only by striking rises in blood pressure but by some decrease in the mortality rate. Withal it must be conceded that there is no overwhelming statistical evidence for the value of these drugs. Only an occasional patient is salvaged.

It is not necessary that all patients with acute myocardial infarction with low blood pressure be treated as if they were in shock. Some of them have been hypotensive for years. There is nothing about the new development of an infarct which would be expected to bring the blood pressure to normal or higher levels. On the other hand, if the previous level of blood pressure is known to have been normal or elevated, and the patient develops an abrupt fall in pressure to 80 or 90 mm. (if previously normal) or to 100 (if previously elevated) and the pressure remains at this new level for an hour or more, he should be treated. If a physician first sees a patient in an acute episode associated with hypotension, and does not know the patient's previous blood pressure level, he can hardly be criticised for treating him for shock. As a general rule, whenever there is any real doubt in the physician's mind, treatment should be given. Patients who are cold, pale and clammy should be treated irrespective of their blood pressure level. On the other hand, patients who look well need not be treated even though their blood pressure is below 90 mm. Apparently there are some patients in whom the severe pain of infarction may produce a fall in blood pressure as a result of peripheral vasodilatation without a fall in cardiac output.[15]

Evidence of vasoconstriction is not a contraindication to the use of pressor substances. The primary change in so-called "cardiogenic shock" is a reduction in the stroke volume output of the left ventricle; the other manifestations are secondary and compensatory mechanisms.[2] Although vasoconstriction is a common feature of spontaneous shock, this constriction is not necessarily maximal. This is attested by appreciable rises in blood pressure which follow the use of pressor amines. At times, a vasoconstrictor mechanism may even be totally lacking; hypotension would be the principal evidence of shock in these patients. There is evidence that the salutary action of the pressor amines is related not only to their effect in elevating the level of blood pressure but also to a direct myocardial effect of these substances. They apparently increase the contractility of the heart and the cardiac output.

Once the existence of shock is established or strongly suspected, treatment should be given forthwith. The longer the duration of the hypotensive state, the greater the likelihood of "shock" entering the "irreversible phase." If the patient is at home, or, if in a hospital, while waiting for an intravenous infusion to be set up, a single dose of Neosynephrine 10–20 mgms., or of Wyamine 35 mgms. is injected intramuscularly. This may be repeated in 15 minutes if ineffective. This is only a temporary expedient since peripheral circulation is decreased and absorption is defective in shock.[16] Hence the intravenous route is vastly to be preferred. An alternative would therefore be the immediate intravenous injection of 20 mgms. of Vasoxyl or 35 mgms. of Wyamine. Meanwhile, 4 cc. of 0.1% Levophed is added to a liter of 5% dextrose in water. Because of the collapsed condition of the veins a "cutdown" may be necessary. The solution is allowed to run into a vein at a rate, generally 20 to 30 drops a minute, sufficient to

elevate the blood pressure to 100 mm. in a previously normo-
tensive person, or to 120 mm. in a previously hypertensive individual, or, most important, to alleviate the manifestations of
shock. This substance has the virtue of increasing coronary
blood flow and the possible disadvantage of decreasing renal
blood flow. In common with most of the newer sympathico-
mimetic amines it has little tendency to induce ectopic rhythms.
When this substance is injected paravenously or subcutaneously it is very prone to produce tissue necrosis. To avoid or
minimize this complication, particularly when prolonged administration seems likely, it is best at the outset to thread a
polyethylene catheter a considerable distance up the vein.
If more concentrated solutions are necessary because of fear
of overloading the circulation in congestive heart failure, or
because of non-responsiveness to the original strength of nor-
epinephrine, this precaution becomes mandatory. Sloughing
frequently occurs despite all efforts at its prevention. A realistic
point of view must be taken in evaluating this risk. In patients
with indubitable shock the immediacy of this shock, and its
implications, much more than overbalance the risk of an even-
tual slough. The latter can generally be dealt with later
utilizing skin grafts if the patient survives. There is evidence
that these sloughs can largely be prevented by the use of
phentolamine (Regitine). The attendant must watch carefully
during and after the infusion of nor-epinephrine for cold,
pale, tender areas along the course of the infusion even if an
intravenous catheter is used. Such areas are infiltrated thoroughly subcutaneously with 5 to 10 cc. of phentolamine and
300 units of hyaluronidase. If the ischemic areas are larger
than 30 cm.² it is recommended [17] that one half of the area be
infiltrated at once and the remaining half 30 minutes later.

In a recent experience with patients in shock it was found
that the addition of phentolamine to the flask of nor-epinephrine eliminated the danger of slough without impairing the

hypertensive effect of the drug. The addition of 5 mgms. of phentolamine to the flask of nor-epinephrine is recommended as adequate to prevent necrosis in areas of extravasation.[18]

Generally if 25 micrograms of Levophed per minute are ineffective, larger doses are not apt to be effective. But one should increase the rate of flow or the strength of the solution to as high as 150 micrograms per minute before concluding that the patient is refractory to the drug.[14] Once an optimal level of blood pressure has been reached and maintained for an hour or two an attempt is made to cut back dosage by slowing the rate of flow. If the blood pressure falls back to or toward the original shock level, the original rate of infusion is restored. Such infusions may be maintained for hours or days. If the blood pressure does not fall on slowing the infusion, further decreases may be attempted. This is the only way to determine the continued need for the drug.

Failure of response may be related, among other causes, to the large size of the infarct and the paucity of remaining healthy myocardium, to inadequate dosage, to pre-existent maximal constriction or to adrenal exhaustion. At times concomitant cortisone therapy, e.g., 150 mgms. by mouth, may render a previously "refractory" patient responsive to this drug.[19] This is true of unresponsiveness to any of the pressor amines and probably indicates impairment of suprarenal function. In a recent case, personally observed, a patient with acute myocardial infarction and pulmonary embolism whose anticoagulant therapy was interrupted for ligation of leg veins, failed to respond to any of an entire series of pressor drugs. Post-mortem examination showed bilateral adrenal hemorrhages, no hemorrhage elsewhere.

My principal experience has been with nor-epinephrine; despite the risk of arrhythmias and sloughing, it remains the choice for definitive treatment. Its use is recommended when shock is full-fledged or where the milder sympathico-mimetic amines have been ineffective. If the patient's condition does not seem so extreme or if there is some doubt about the true existence of shock, the tendency will be to use the milder vasopressor drugs. Neosynephrine, 50 to 100 mgms. in 1000 cc. of dextrose in water may be given in the same manner as nor-epinephrine. Vasoxyl is available for intravenous or intramuscular use in 1 cc. ampoules each containing 20 mgms. At first this may be tried undiluted in doses of 10, 15 or 20 mgms. If necessary this may be given as often as four times an hour. If a single dose of 40 mgms. is ineffective, the use of this substance should be abandoned. Once effectiveness has been demonstrated, a smoother effect of longer duration can be achieved by giving it by continuous intravenous infusion. For this purpose the contents of two ampoules are added to 250 cc. of 5% dextrose in water. Wyamine, 35 to 70 mgms., diluted in 100 cc. of 5% glucose solution may be given by slow intravenous drip at the rate of approximately 1 mgm. per minute. Aramine in the strength of 50 to 200 mgms. dissolved in 1000 cc. of 5% dextrose solution is given at the rate of 2 to 6 cc. per minute. Ephedrine sulfate 35 to 50 mgms. dissolved in 100 cc. of dextrose in water may be infused intravenously in the manner described for nor-epinephrine. An effective blood pressure level may also be maintained by intramuscular injections of 25 mgms. of ephedrine every hour or two. With all of these substances it is necessary that dosage be titrated continuously utilizing the general plan outlined above in the discussion of nor-epinephrine. To regulate dosage corresponding to the changing needs of the patient and to guard against para-venous injection, the infusion must be constantly monitored by a physician or nurse.

These materials may not always be at hand. But most physicians carry a supply of epinephrine in their bags. This may be given by hypodermic injection in the dose of 0.3 to 0.5 cc. of a 1:1000 solution and rationed at appropriate intervals determined by the response of the patient. Or epinephrine may be given by vein in the manner described under the treatment of Stokes-Adams attacks (p. 299). This drug, of course, has a much greater tendency than nor-epinephrine, and certainly than any of the milder vasopressors, to accelerate the heart and induce arrhythmias. In shock associated with complete heart block Isuprel or epinephrine will be the drug of choice.

DIGITALIS

Although digitalis has long been regarded as dangerous in shock and to be avoided at all costs, recent speculation [20] and limited clinical experience [21] suggest that this group of drugs may at times actually have a salutary, or even a dramatic, effect. The purpose of the drug is to increase the stroke work of the heart and thus the perfusion pressure and minute volume output of the heart.[21] Digitalis would certainly be indicated where there is frank evidence of congestive heart failure. But even if evidence of failure is lacking, a favorable effect may be obtained. It has been suggested that digitalis may potentiate the action of vasopressor drugs. Digitalis must be given most cautiously. In a previously undigitalized patient, Digoxin may be injected intravenously in a dose of 0.5 to 1.0 mgm. over the course of five minutes as an initial dose. It may be justifiable also to use digitalis in patients who have not responded to other measures. The situation here is a most desperate one and desperation measures may be justifiable. In the difficult therapeutic dilemma presented by the patient in both shock and congestive heart failure, another gamble beside digitalization may be lifesaving, particularly if the patient is orthopneic; this is phlebotomy.[22] But the physician must be prepared [22] to retransfuse all or part of the blood in the event of the patient's deterioration.

[46]

The shock of myocardial infarction presents a special problem, that of maintaining an adequate pressure head through the coronary arteries. In this emergency the demands made of therapy are thus more rigorous than in other medical conditions associated with shock. We have therefore not hesitated to use the pressor amines in the shock of mesenteric embolism, pulmonary embolism or of congestive heart failure itself. Where there is associated evidence of, or the likelihood of, blood loss, as in the shock attending dissecting aneurysm of the aorta or in patients with gastrointestinal hemorrhage complicated by myocardial infarction, transfusion is necessary.

Shock may be the prime evidence for the development of an arrhythmia, e.g., atrial fibrillation or flutter or paroxysmal ventricular tachycardia. It is not rare for a patient to come out of shock immediately on reversion to normal sinus rhythm. An arrhythmia may, on the other hand, be a complication of shock, a complication which is to be treated but whose successful termination will not be followed by disappearance of shock. If control of a known arrhythmia has no effect on shock, one should suspect another underlying cause. Thus in one recently observed patient shock persisted though flutter was controlled. This was due to the undetected and concealed bleeding of a duodenal ulcer.

REFERENCES

(1) Selzer, A.: The hypotensive state following acute myocardial infarction. I. Clinical observations. Am. Ht. J. *44*: 1, 1952.
(2) Freis, E. D., Schnaper, H. W., Johnson, R. L. and Schreiner, G. E.: Hemodynamic alterations in acute myocardial infarction. I. Cardiac output, mean arterial pressure, total peripheral resistance, "central" and total

blood volumes, venous pressure and average circulation time. J.C.I. *31*:131, 1952.

(3) Corday, E., Bergman, H. C., Schwartz, L. L., Spritzler, R. J. and Prinzmetal, M.: Studies on the coronary circulation. IV. The effect of shock on the heart and its treatment. Am. Ht. J. *37*: 560, 1949.

(4) Sampson, J. J. and Singer, I. M.: Plasma and blood infusion following myocardial infarction. Am. Ht. J. *38*: 54, 1949.

(5) Epstein, F. H. and Relman, A. S.: Transfusion treatment of shock due to myocardial infarction. N.E.J. Med. *241*: 889, 1949.

(6) Berman, E. F. and Akman, L. C.: Intra-arterial infusion in the treatment of shock resulting from coronary occlusion. Am. Ht. J. *43*: 264, 1952.

(7) Case, R. B., Sarnoff, S. J., Waithe, P. E. and Sarnoff, L. C.: Intra-arterial and intravenous blood infusion in hemorrhagic shock. Comparison of effects on coronary blood flow and arterial pressure. J.A.M.A. *152*: 208, 1953.

(8) Kurland, G. S. and Malach, M.: The clinical use of norepinephrine in the treatment of shock accompanying myocardial infarction and other conditions. N.E.J. Med. *247*: 383, 1952.

(9) Fink, T. R., d'Angio, C. J. and Biloon, S.: Clinical study of shock following myocardial infarction. J.A.M.A. *151*: 1163, 1953.

(10) Hellerstein, H. K., Brofman, B. L. and Caskey, W. H.: Shock accompanying myocardial infarction: treatment with pressor amines. Am. Ht. J. *44*: 407, 1952.

(11) Nathanson, M. H. and Miller, H.: Clinical observations on a new epinephrine-like compound, methoxamine. Am. J. Med. Sci. *223*: 270, 1952.

(12) Moyer, J. H. and Beazley, H. L.: Effectiveness of Aramine in the treatment of shock. Am. Ht. J. *50*: 136, 1955.

(13) Miller, A. J. and Baker, L. A.: L-arterenol (Levophed) in the treatment of shock due to acute myocardial infarction. Arch. Int. Med. 89: 591, 1952.

(14) Sampson, J. J. and Zipser, A.: Nor-epinephrine in shock following myocardial infarction. Influence upon survival rate and renal function. Circulation 9: 38, 1954.

(15) Lee, G. Quoted in reference 21.

(16) Hellerstein, H. K. and Brofman, B. L.: The treatment of the hypotensive state accompanying myocardial infarction. Modern Concepts of Cardiovascular Disease. 20: 104, 1951.

(17) Close, A. S.: Phenoltamine hydrochloride in prevention of cutaneous necrosis due to levarterenol. J.A.M.A. *170*: 1916, 1959.

(18) Zucker, G., Eisinger, R. P., Floch, M. H. and Singer, M. M.: Prevention of ischemic necrosis by use of levarterenol-phentolamine mixtures in treatment of shock. Proc. 32nd Scientific Sessions Am. Ht. Ass'n., Oct. 23–25, 1959, p. 789.

(19) Kurland, G. S. and Freedberg, A. S.: Potentiating effect of ACTH and cortisone on pressor response to intravenous infusion of l-nor-epinephrine. Proc. Soc. Exper. Biol. and Med. 78: 28, 1951.

(20) Boyer, N. H.: Digitalis in acute myocardial infarction. N.E.J. Med. 252: 536, 1955.

(21) Gorlin, R. and Robin, E. D.: Cardiac glycosides in the treatment of cardiogenic shock. Brit. Med. J. *1*: 937, 1955.

(22) Stead, E. A., Jr. and Ebert, R. V.: Shock syndrome produced by failure of the heart. Arch. Int. Med. 69: 369, 1942.

3

CARDIOGENIC CHEST PAIN —

THE CORONARY

EMERGENCIES

Angina Pectoris

Coronary Insufficiency

Acute Myocardial Infarction

Intravenous Therapy in Coronary Artery Disease

"Arm-Chair" Treatment

Anticoagulant Therapy

3

CARDIOGENIC CHEST PAIN —

THE CORONARY

EMERGENCIES

Whether or not its cause has been determined, pain in the chest may constitute an acute emergency. In many cases pain in the chest is due to disease in extrathoracic or in intrathoracic but extracardiac structures. But much more often than not, particularly in middle age, such pain is the consequence of heart disease. Pain resulting from coronary artery disease is customarily classified in three categories arranged in order of increasing gravity: angina pectoris, "coronary insufficiency" ("coronary failure") and acute myocardial infarction. It is generally considered that this pain somehow arises in consequence of myocardial hypoxia.

ANGINA PECTORIS

The least of these disturbances is angina pectoris. Its clinical features are too well known to deserve description here. The most striking feature in the examination of a patient during a paroxysm is his immobility and incommunicability. His heart rate may be normal or accelerated. The blood pressure is characteristically higher than it is when he is free of this pain. He may hold his hand over the front of his chest, frequently in a characteristic clenching gesture. He tends involuntarily to assume the same attitude in later describing his discomfort. This sign may be equally helpful in articulate and inarticulate individuals. After the subsidence of an attack examination may be quite negative. It is from the history, and not from the examination, that the diagnosis should be made. The electrocardiogram may or may not show evidence of pre-existent heart disease. A tracing recorded during the actual symptoms may be of greater value, showing in certain leads depression of the RS-T segments characteristic of subendocardial ischemia. Another feature of this condition is its prompt relief by nitroglycerin; to a greater or lesser extent this may thus have diagnostic as well as therapeutic value. If the physician slows the patient's heart by stimulating his carotid sinus, a decision can often be made whether this discomfort is coronary in origin. If the patient indicates that he is having pain which is identical with that of his presenting complaint, and if his heart is slowed appreciably by this maneuver, one should ask whether the chest discomfort has become worse. If the patient replies that, on the contrary, it has disappeared, one may assume that the discomfort is the result of coronary impairment.[3] This, then, confirms the diagnosis of angina pectoris. Some patients find, on their own accord, that taking a deep breath relieves the symptoms; it is possible that this depends upon a similar slowing mechanism.

There are two circumstances when the pain of angina pectoris may take on the aspect of a cardiac emergency. The first is when this pain is a new and terrifying experience to the patient and its cause has not yet been determined. Upon repetition of the paroxysm and recognition of its transient nature the patient need not regard it with the same alarm. The second is when measures used in its management of themselves give rise to disturbing side-effects.

Far and away the most effective treatment of angina pectoris is the use of nitroglycerin. This is preferably prescribed as the hypodermic tablet in the dose of 0.3 mgm. This is placed under the tongue where it is allowed to dissolve. This generally requires 10 to 20 seconds. If the tablet triturate is used, its disintegration may be hastened by sucking the tablet or grinding it up with the teeth. Its absorption is indicated by a sense of flushing or fullness in the head or by a severe expanding headache. Sometimes the latter symptoms are so severe that the patient feels that the headache is worse than the chest pain and he is discouraged from the further use of the medication. Hence it is desirable to start with small doses and, if necessary, to work up to larger doses. If a tablet of certain size induces headache, the patient should be instructed to break the tablet approximately in half and use the half tablet for subsequent chest pain. Tablets containing as little as 0.15 mgm. or even 0.12 mgm. are available. Some patients who develop headache are not particularly disturbed by it and are willing to use nitroglycerin in spite of this side-effect. Others appear to develop this untoward effect on any dose of the drug however small. Many patients, feeling that the use of the drug may be a sign of moral softness or that in time it may be followed by intolerance or habituation, are reluctant to use nitroglycerin. If they are convinced that it is really effective in aborting the pain, these patients should be encouraged to use it.

In rare instances, nitroglycerin induces cardiovascular collapse.[4,5,6] Such reactions appear to be more common in hypertensive women and are more prone to occur in the upright than the recumbent position.[6] I recall one hypertensive patient who had an attack of angina pectoris while I was examining her. This was relieved by nitroglycerin. While being fluoroscoped shortly thereafter, she broke out in a cold sweat and slumped to the floor. Her blood pressure was found to have fallen to extremely low levels. Another patient, likewise hypertensive, awoke with pain at 2 in the morning, took a nitroglycerin tablet from the bedside table and was relieved of his pain. He then felt that, as long as he was awake, he might as well get up. A little while later he fell to the bathroom floor while urinating ("Micturition syncope"). It is of interest that each of these instances of nitroglycerin collapse occurred when the patient took the medication while reclining or sitting, then got up into an immobile upright position shortly afterward. It has been shown experimentally that vasomotor collapse induced by the prototype of nitroglycerin, sodium nitrite, depends upon the combined effect of nitrite and tilting.[7,8] I have seen one patient in whom nitroglycerin was generally effective in relieving her angina. On three occasions, however, it induced severe faintness and sweating; each of these occured a long time, four or five hours, after a meal. The possibility exists here of enhancement of this nitroglycerin effect by hypoglycemia. There are indeed rare patients in whom angina pectoris itself seems to be triggered by hypoglycemia.[9,10] These may be helped by having the patient swallow hard candy, or prevented by having him on a high protein diet.

One virtue of nitroglycerin is that it may be taken relatively inconspicuously. The inhalation of amyl nitrite from a perle crushed in a handkerchief or of octyl nitrite from an inhaler (Medi-haler-Nitro) is not to be recommended. This has the disadvantage of presenting the patient with varying doses of the active substances and of making therapy, though effective, embarrassingly conspicuous. It is this desire for unobtrusiveness that explains why so many patients with angina pectoris are content merely to stop and suffer it out while pretending to look up an address or while shifting something from one pocket to another or gazing admiringly into a store window. Amyl nitrite, furthermore, has a characteristic and easily identified pungent odor.

Generally, if one nitroglycerin table is ineffective, a second may be taken in the same way as the first. If this too is ineffective the patient may be one of the small number of people with classical angina pectoris who simply do not respond to nitroglycerin. Or his pain may be due to some cause other than angina pectoris, for example, myocardial infarction. It is important to remember that nitroglycerin may also be effective in relieving pain due to smooth muscle spasm elsewhere; the pain of esophageal spasm or gall bladder disease, for example, may likewise be terminated. A number of my patients, some of them otherwise teetotalers, are convinced that a small whiskey or brandy is more effective than nitroglycerin in relieving their pain. This salutary effect of alcohol, well-known to Osler and Harlow Brooks,[11] apparently depends upon its effect on the central nervous system rather than on coronary blood flow.[12,13] Erythrol tetranitrate (Erythrityl Tetranitrate) is almost as effective as nitroglycerin when taken sublingually; its effect is more prolonged than that of nitroglycerin. Mention has already been made of the carotid sinus stimulation test for coronary insufficiency. This procedure may also have therapeutic usefulness. Patients with known angina pectoris, in whom carotid sinus stimulation consistently slows the heart, may predictably be relieved of individual paroxysms by this maneuver. This may be done by physician or patient, taking the precautions described on pages 204 and 205.

It goes almost without saying that the angina pectoris which is due to or triggered by some underlying condition such as thyrotoxicosis, aortic valve disease, paroxysmal rapid heart action of one type or another, or hemorrhage, should be treated by appropriate means, even if one suspects that in most of these cases there must be an important degree of coronary artery disease as well. Specific precipitating factors such as going out of doors in the cold immediately after meals or walking briskly upgrade should be avoided. Warming the air by breathing through a muffler or taking nitroglycerin prophylactically may be worth-while. And there is a definite place in the treatment of angina pectoris with sedative or tranquilizing agents.

At times, angina pectoris occurs on the very slightest exertion or at rest. It may occur in this way repeatedly throughout the day, always responding to nitroglycerin. But no sooner is one paroxysm aborted than another sets in. It may thus be present almost constantly during the day. Here, nitroglycerin, given as directed above, is the first choice in therapy. There is little doubt of its effectiveness. But the drug has to be given repeatedly, at times as often as 40 times a day. These patients may be assured that, since the effect of the drug is disseminated rapidly without cumulative effect, this practice is not dangerous. The drug may be taken for pain anticipated as well as for pain already in progress.

CORONARY INSUFFICIENCY

There is a group of patients whose symptomatology is intermediate between that of angina pectoris and that of cardiac infarction.[1,2,14,15] Their pain is more prolonged than that of angina pectoris. It is not relieved characteristically by nitroglycerin. But they have little if any evidence of tissue breakdown. The temperature, white blood count, sedimentation rate and lactic acid dehydrogenase or transaminase remain normal. If complicated by myocardial necrosis these parameters may be abnormal. The electrocardiogram may show no changes at all or it may develop changes in the RS-T segments or in the T waves; but changes diagnostic of myocardial infarction do not appear. In many respects the treatment of coronary insufficiency is more difficult than that of actual myocardial infarction.

Where the coronary insufficiency is secondary to some remediable condition such as paroxysmal tachycardia, gastrointestinal bleeding, shock, acute pulmonary embolism or infection, appropriate treatment, be it quinidine, transfusion, Levophed, anticoagulant or antibiotic, is mandatory.[15] Allaying the patient's fear that he is actually suffering a heart attack is often very helpful. Much more important than any of the numerous medications which have been recommended for this condition is the prescription of a period of two or three weeks of rest in the form of a modified "coronary regimen" in chair or bed away from telephone and visitors. In some patients this is best carried out in the hospital, in others, especially where the expense of hospitalization would be unduly burdensome, at home. For some reason, presumably because of the restoration of an adequate blood supply to regions of the heart whose previous irrigation was tenuous, these patients may in time lose their continuous pain. It is not uncommon to see patients, desperately ill with coronary insufficiency, angina decubitus or status anginosus, in whom no medication whatever seemed to be effective and for whom various forms of surgery have been contemplated, who have somehow, after such a period of rest, proceeded to carry on very well, even as breadwinners, over a period of years.

Nitroglycerin may be given liberally and, if effective, repetitively, but morphine or meperidine (Demerol), given in the manner described below under acute myocardial infarction, may be necessary to control the initial pain. Just as soon as milder analgesics can be utilized effectively the physician must discontinue these narcotics. This is not always an easy matter, for the conscientious physician may be hard put to decide how much the patient's complaints are due to real pain and how much to a conscious or unconscious desire for the pleasant euphoria conferred by either drug. Certain it is that a respectable proportion of Demerol addiction has its roots in the soil of refractory coronary insufficiency. At this time, too, it seems to me that it is best to avoid the use of alcohol.

A course of heparin therapy given in a dose of 50 to 100 mgms. intramuscularly once or twice a week has been reported as quite effective against the pain of coronary insufficiency.[16] A favorable response to this substance could be related to its anticoagulant effect, to its effect as a clearing agent against neutral fat in the serum, to an increase in coronary blood flow or perhaps to a specific effect against the pain of coronary artery disease. My experience with this form of treatment has been unimpressive. And it has been reported [17] as without significant effect upon the electrocardiographic response to standard exercise. Coronary insufficiency should always be regarded as a possible precursor to, or possibly an incipient phase of, actual myocardial infarction. In the original experimental observations on the value of anticoagulant therapy against myocardial infarction it was heparin that was studied, and it was in precisely such a preventive, not curative, fashion that it was employed.[18] The question has recently been raised whether dicumarol too might have a direct pain-relieving effect. There is as yet no convincing evidence that dicumarol or heparin, given in the stage of coronary insufficiency, will, in a significant proportion of cases, prevent the materialization of actual infarction. Certainly many patients who seem to be headed in this direction have gone on to infarction in spite of optimal dicumarol effect upon the prothrombin time or optimal heparin effect upon the clotting time. For coronary insufficiency refractory to the above measures a number of medications and surgical procedures of doubtful or unproven merit are available for trial. But these are not emergency measures and will not be discussed in this treatise. It seems rational to try these individually and in series and by "trial and error" rather than more than one at a time. It seems wise also to continue with whatever seems to be effective even though one may have personal doubts that this is actually as effective as it seems.

Numerous instances of coronary insufficiency have appeared actually to have been initiated during, if not by, hypotensive therapy. This includes rauwolfia preparations, Apresoline, Ansolysen and Diuril. Their continued use can hardly be recommended under these circumstances. Furthermore, if the patient has been receiving maintenance thyroid therapy, given for whatever purpose, this should be discontinued at once on the development of coronary insufficiency.

ACUTE MYOCARDIAL INFARCTION

A detailed recital of the signs and symptoms of acute myocardial infarction would be superfluous here. But a few words may be in order regarding the laboratory substantiation of this diagnosis. The temperature, the white blood cell count or the sedimentation rate, alone or in combination, may be significantly elevated. Certain enzymes, such as transaminase or lactic acid dehydrogenase, may be measured in the blood serum in higher than normal concentration. These changes may be detected early in the course of the acute episode or only after the lapse of two, three or more days. The electrocardiogram may show characteristic changes, including elevation of the RS-T segments, inversion of the T waves or the development of broad, prominent Q or QS waves where such changes do not belong, all of these electrical phenomena developing in a dynamic sequence. These changes may begin at the very onset or only after several days or even weeks—or not at all. Where these signs are absent it is mandatory to repeat these tests at frequent intervals, daily in the case of the white count and sedimentation rate, four-hourly (generally omitting sleeping hours) and rectally in the case of the temperature, and every two or three days in the case of the electrocardiogram. Once definite evidence of tissue breakdown or diagnostic electrocardiographic changes have been demonstrated there is no point to willy-nilly repetition of these tests. The order for daily laboratory work should be discontinued and the temperature should now be taken by mouth and only four times a day. The common practice of routine hourly or two-hourly blood pressure determinations around the clock is superfluous and deprives the patient of badly needed rest. In the absence of a definite indication, such as an undefined arrhythmia, there is no need to repeat the electrocardiogram at frequent intervals. The excuse is frequently offered that this is important in detecting extension of the infarct. Actually the electrocardiogram is helpful in this way in only the most unusual circumstances. The clinical development of renewed chest pain or sweating or shock are much more helpful in directing suspicion to this possibility. Those electrocardiographic changes which are detected in the absence of such clinical clues are at best of dubious significance. A single repeat tracing is justifiable at the time of the discharge of the patient from the hospital or from the physician's care.

It goes without saying that one does not wait for a definite diagnosis before helping the patient with chest pain. When seen as an acute emergency, the complaint is ordinarily of moderately or excruciatingly severe pain. One is satisfied with an adequate history and physical examination, omitting such details as family history, habits, ophthalmoscopic, otoscopic, rectal or pelvic examination. A complete and exhausting physical examination at this time merely gives a false aura of scientific thoroughness; worse than this, it is inhumane.

In the absence of such contraindication as the pulmonocardiac failure of patients with important chest deformities, morphine is the drug of choice. This may be given subcutaneously in a dose of 10 to 15 mgms. or, rarely, intravenously, in a dose of 4 to 8 mgms. The initial subcutaneous dose may be repeated every fifteen or twenty minutes until a total of 60 mgms. is given over the course of an hour or even 120 mgms. in two hours. Such large doses are only very rarely necessary. Yet the amount of drug that may be taken during severe pain without the development of toxic symptoms is phenomenal compared with the amount that would be an overdose were the patient free of pain. It is incumbent upon the physician to remain with the patient until his pain is relieved. There are some patients in whom morphine induces severe vomiting. Where this sensitivity is already known, the physician will prefer some other analgesic agent. The act of vomiting may be an undesirable physical strain at this time. Following an injection of morphine, the physician may not know whether the vomiting is the result of the acute infarct as such or of the medication. And the patient will probably become constipated in a day or two after the injection. When it is not known whether the patient is sensitive to the drug, the physician may take his chances with morphine in spite of these possibilities. Many physicians use a hypodermic tablet containing a combination of morphine and atropine. This is a satisfactory combination for preoperative use but there is no good evidence that atropine is helpful as an adjunct in the relief of the pain of myocardial infarction.

In case of sensitivity to morphine, meperidine hydrochloride (Demerol) 50 to 75 mgms. may be given hypodermically. The theoretic objection has been raised that this drug has a very mild vagolytic (parasympathicolytic) effect and thus would accelerate the heart rate. I have never been impressed with this and have employed the drug without hesitation and with good effect. An alternative narcotic preparation for hypodermic administration is dihydromorphinone hydrochloride (Dilaudid) 2 to 4 mgms. Papaverine, which is quite devoid of narcotic action, has no place in the relief of the pain of myocardial infarction. In an uncomplicated attack of acute myocardial infarction it is only rarely necessary to continue the use of any of these narcotic agents beyond the initial episode of pain. One need, in fact, have no fear of continuing the use of these preparations as often as is necessary for pain during the first few days. Occasionally it is necessary to continue with some milder analgesic but generally it is possible to discontinue all narcotics and analgesics, perhaps continuing with some mild sedative, for the next few days. As indicated above, the problem of addiction is much more likely to develop in patients with prolonged coronary insufficiency than in acute myocardial infarction. In the latter condition the patient usually has his pain, then gets over it.

Many of the narcotic preparations are available as a tablet which must be dissolved and prepared for hypodermic injection. This is a very fussy and time-consuming procedure. A teaspoon, hypodermic syringe and needle are boiled in an inch or so of water in a small dipper. Time can be saved by asking, at the time of the telephone call, for someone in the family to have the water boiling while awaiting the arrival of the physician. The syringe and needle are assembled aseptically. The spoon, containing boiled water, is removed from the dipper and placed in a stable position. Water is drawn into the syringe, the hypodermic tablet placed in the still uncontaminated spoon and the hot water irrigated back and forth until the tablet is entirely dissolved. Its disintegration may be hurried by breaking it up with the needle. Many of these preparations are available ready dissolved in an ampoule or vial. Used with a disposable-ready-sterilized syringe (Hypack, Discardit) or with an autoclaved syringe carried in a metal tube from the physician's bag, the medication can be given much more promptly. It should be the responsibility of the physician or his nurse to be certain that an adequate supply of sterilized hypo-kits are in his bag. In a pinch one can sterilize syringe and needle by irrigating them with rubbing alcohol, drawing the narcotic from the alcohol-sponged vial or ampoule and injecting. I have never seen infection follow this practice.

INTRAVENOUS THERAPY IN CORONARY ARTERY DISEASE

A word about the intravenous injection of these substances. In general this is only very rarely necessary. When the pain is truly agonizing this route may be employed. But partial to complete relief follows quite rapidly—in 20 minutes or so—in most cases when the medication is given hypodermically. Where these drugs are given intravenously almost as a routine, one cannot help but wonder to what extent this is for the patient's and to what extent for the physician's or the family's benefit.

Many observers have felt that in patients with coronary artery disease there may be a distinct vulnerability to coronary pain or myocardial infarction on the intravenous injection of foreign substances. I first became interested in this possibility during the era of serum therapy for lobar pneumonia when a patent with an old myocardial infarct succumbed about a half hour after an initial injection of Type I pneumococcal anti-serum. The manner of her death was cardiac, not respiratory. All recommended precautions as to pre-testing, rate of infusion, temperature and clarity of the solution had been meticulously observed. Shortly after this a case was reported[19] of a man with angina pectoris who developed Type VIII pneumococcus pneumonia and complained of squeezing chest pain after each of four doses of specific anti-serum. Following the fifth dose he suddenly expired. Post-mortem examination showed old and fresh myocardial infarction. In addition to specific anti-serum of various types, fatal, or near-fatal, reactions have followed the intravenous injection of mercurial diuretics,[20] aminophylline,[21,22] diodrast[23] and sodium tetra-iodo-phenolpathalein.[24] The mechanism of these reactions may differ from case to case. They may be due to a specific toxic effect upon the myocardium[20] in some instances, to allergic reactions in

[65]

others,[25,26] to the speed of infusion in some cases,[22] to a shock-like lowering of the systemic pressure and consequent inadequate coronary irrigation [14,19] in others and, perhaps in a few, to a peculiar vulnerability of the coronary arteries.

It is very difficult to be sure of a cause and effect relationship. So many people with heart disease, with a certain proportion inexorably destined to catastrophic complication, receive so many injections for so many purposes and on so many occasions, that it is inevitable that a certain number of severe reactions or even fatalities should develop after injections. These reactions must represent an extremely small proportion of the total number of injections given these patients. Nevertheless the conscientious physician, the man at the barrel end of the syringe, who sees such a reaction occur immediately after his injection cannot help but feel, as did one of the above [24] that "the development of the infarct was so striking as to leave in the minds of those who watched the episode a fixed impression that the injection of foreign material into the circulation of this patient had in some fashion precipitated an occlusion of one of the coronary arteries."

Entirely aside from any specific chemical or immunologic property of its contents, the volume, tonicity and rate of injection of solutions is important. The danger of intravenous fluid injections comes when large volumes of fluid are given too rapidly to a patient with an unrecognized cardiac defect.[28,29] It seems wise, therefore, to regard parenteral therapy as potentially dangerous in patients with coronary artery disease. In the absence of a definite reason to the contrary it is wise to medicate such a patient by mouth rather than parenterally and hypodermically rather than intravenously, and, where intravenous infusion is necessary, slowly rather than rapidly.

There are a few patients who concede that oxygen has actually allayed the severity of the pain of their myocardial infarction. My experience has been that oxygen is ineffective as a pain reliever in this condition. This is anticipated by the demonstration that 100% oxygen does not alleviate the electro-cardiographic response to standard exercise of patients with angina pectoris.[30] This is not to say that it should not be used in myocardial infarction, if other conditions, such as severe dyspnea, pulmonary congestion or edema exist. One very important reason for withholding oxygen therapy is this: it is all too apt to impress the patient with the seriousness of his condition and even to terrify him. Certainly if, for any reason, the patient resists the idea of oxygen, one should not persist in its use.

Failure of relief by nitroglycerin is one of the features which distinguishes the pain of acute myocardial infarction from that of angina pectoris. It is commonly taught that once it has been proved that one or two nitroglycerin tablets are ineffective, particularly if this medication has been effective in the same patient for antecedent angina pectoris, the further use of this substance is potentially dangerous.[31] It is reasoned that, by significantly lowering systemic blood pressure, it might further embarrass coronary perfusion. Such a policy seems wise during the initial episode of pain. With recurrent pain following the initial crisis, however, it has been my experience that nitroglycerin is frequently effective and I can recommend cautious trial with this drug as well worth the effort. I have seen no harm and much good come of this practice.

At times, the precordial infiltration of 0.5% solution of procaine will relieve the pain of acute myocardial infarction. One need not be apprehensive about the minute amounts of epinephrine which are generally contained in the solution of this anesthetic agent to localize its effect.

"ARM CHAIR" TREATMENT

Starting as early as the first or second day, so long as he is not in shock, the patient with acute myocardial infarction should be out of bed, seated in a well-padded chair, for as many hours of the day as he will tolerate. The rationale and details of the "arm chair" treatment are given on pages 137 to 140.

ANTICOAGULANT THERAPY

The application of any measure which achieves a reduction in the mortality rate of acute myocardial infarction from 23 to 16%,[32] must be viewed as an emergency measure even though the effects of this treatment are not immediately apparent. Most observers are agreed that anticoagulant therapy is worthwhile from the standpoint of the total group afflicted with acute myocardial infraction. But some feel that it is possible to select at the outset of their attack good risk patients who need not be treated since they will do well anyway. Others feel less confident of their skill at anticipating the course which a given patient will follow and, therefore, treat all indiscriminately.

My own practice is to treat with anticoagulants all patients in whom a definite diagnosis has been made and in whom no contraindication exists. If the patient is first observed at the outset of his attack he is started on dicumarol or coumadin; if first seen after the second day he is given both heparin, for its immediate effect, and either dicumarol or coumadin, for its late developing effect. Once an optimal prothrombin time has been attained heparin is discontinued.

Anticoagulant therapy should not be employed in patients with liver disease associated with spontaneous hypoprothrombinemia, in those with certain blood dyscrasias, or with a bleeding tendency from any cause or in patients with hematuria or melena. It should be avoided in those giving a history of peptic ulcer, certainly if the ulcer has ever bled. Other contraindications would be recent surgery on the brain, spinal cord, joints, genitourinary tract or any surgery where large raw areas are left or where concealed hemorrhage can occur.

There are two principal classes of anticoagulants. The first of these is heparin. It must be given parenterally. Its effect is rapid in development, is gauged by measurement of the clotting time and is readily and rapidly abolished by protamine. The other is the coumarin and the inanedione derivatives. These are effective by mouth. Their effect, as measured by the prothrombin time, is slower in development and more reluctantly antagonized by Vitamin K_1 oxide. Heparin is expensive; coumarin and inanedione compounds are relatively inexpensive.

When an immediate or prompt anticoagulant effect is desired, as when treatment is started after the third or fourth day of an attack of acute myocardial infarction, or when there is difficulty with veins so that frequent venipuncture for prothrombin time will be impossible, heparin should be used. For immediate effect heparin is given by deep intramuscular injection or by subcutaneous injection, using a small needle, in the dose of 50 mgms. every six hours, varying dosage or interval in accordance with the clotting time. A convenient schedule would be 6 A.M., 12 noon, 6 P.M. and 12 midnight. A "five-hour clotting time," done only on the first day or two of treatment, should be between 25 and 40 minutes. Such an effect can be anticipated within a half-hour of the initial injection. If veins are no longer accessible, heparin may be given in an arbitrary schedule in the Swedish fashion[33] giving 150 mgms. as an initial dose, repeated at four-hourly intervals during the first day of treatment; then on the following days four injections daily, each of 100 mgms. Depo-heparin is painful, continuous intravenous heparin infusion difficult. Some of the newer preparations are not painful. Lipo-hepin may be injected with a tuberculin syringe and 25 gauge needle in the amount of 0.1 cc. or 0.2 cc. subcutaneously into a fold of the abdominal skin. Injections can be given twice daily tattooing sequentially across the abdomen, somewhat as the site of insulin injections is rotated.

In the event of hemorrhage it may be necessary to abolish the anticoagulant effect of heparin. This may be achieved by calculating the probable amount of heparin in the body on the basis of the previous dose of heparin, making allowance for excretion. One then substitutes milligram of protamine for estimated milligram of heparin and injects this amount by vein. The effect of this amount of protamine is then checked by the clotting time and further increments given if necessary.

Where the need for anticoagulant effect is not immediate, one may proceed more leisurely, using one of the coumarin or inanedione derivatives. Generally it is wise, in view of the possibility of spontaneous hypoprothrombinemia, to measure the prothrombin time before any of these compounds is given. In very rare instances it may be justifiable to initiate therapy with these hypoprothrombinemic agents when an initial prothrombin time cannot be measured, for example, "after hours" or on a week-end when a reliable technician may not be available; the risk that there may be an unrecognized spontaneous hypoprothrombinemia must then be deliberately assumed.

Probably the most widely used of the coumarin compounds is dicumarol.[34] This is given in an initial dose of 300 mgms. by mouth, assuming an initial prothrombin time (P.T.) between 75 and 100% concentration. If this has dropped by the second day to, say, 50%, an additional 150 to 200 mgms. may be given. On the third day and thereafter it is necessary to juggle the dosage, aiming at keeping the P.T. between 10 and 25%. There is no set dosage; perhaps 25 mgms. per day would be an average dose but this must be determined every day, or, later on, perhaps every other day, by measurement of the P.T. Generally an optimal level is not attained until the third, occasionally not until the fifth or sixth day.

Excessive hypoprothrombinemia is a calculated risk in anticoagulant therapy with these compounds. The opinion has been expressed that, since hemorrhage from excessive dosage is merely an extension of the pharmacological effect of the drug, it should be regarded as a complication, not as a toxic effect. Such a contention seems specious and the distinction a semantic one. Whether a toxic effect or a complication, hemorrhage is the most frequent and most feared development during treatment with these drugs. If the prothrombin time falls below 10% the next daily dose of the drug is omitted. It is not always necessary to give Vitamin K or Vitamin K_1 oxide (phytonedione), but if the level falls below 5% or if, after the drug has been omitted, the concentration does not return toward the original level during the ensuing day, Mephyton should be given by mouth in the dose of 5 to 10 mgms. If the patient has shown gross clinical or occult laboratory evidence of bleeding (ecchymoses, epistaxis, melena, gross or microscopic hematuria), Mephyton emulsion should be given very slowly by vein in the dose of 50 mgms. of the drug. This injection may be accompanied or followed by excruciating flank pain, reminiscent of that occurring in dissecting aneurysm, but the pain generally subsides in 20 minutes or so. It has been recommended [35] that if the resumption of coumarin compounds is contemplated or anticipated, it is desirable to avoid too drastic a dose of Vitamin K_1 oxide else the patient becomes refractory to further anticoagulant effect for periods up to five days. It is my practice, unless my hand is forced back to the use of anticoagulants, rather to abandon this form of therapy altogether once hemorrhagic complications develop. Transfusions, preferably of fresh blood, may be necessary or imperative at the same time for uncontrolled bleeding.

Blood for the determination of the prothrombin time is drawn early in the morning and the determination run promptly, preferably within four hours. If it is impossible to run the test promptly the plasma should be centrifuged off immediately after the blood is obtained. The result of the test is generally known by noon. The dose is given in capsule form at bedtime. This facilitates uniform absorption. In my experience it has been impossible to maintain the prothrombin time uniformly within the optimal 10 to 25% range with dicumarol. One of the reasons for "escape" in either direction is probably the "give and take" of bowel absorption.

It is important that, insofar as possible, the prothrombin test be performed by the same experienced technician throughout the week. Another common cause of the "escapes" mentioned above is the unavailability of this person at all times. Week-end prothrombin times done by a medical student, interne or physician who is otherwise engaged during the remainder of the week, are generally unreliable. This is not an appropriate place for a detailed description of the technique of measuring the prothrombin time. The reader will note that in this discussion the results are expressed in terms of per cent, imparting an aura of super-scientific accuracy to the determination. Actually this is merely the preference and custom of the group with whom I have worked. To determine the per cent, the test is done in exactly the same manner as the measurement of actual time. Then depending upon the prothrombin time of a normal individual determined that same morning, one derives, with the aid of an appropriate conversion chart (Fig. 5) the corresponding percentage. Thus if the control plasma had a prothrombin time of 14 seconds (dotted line), while the "unknown" had a time of 27 seconds (ordinate), the prothrombin time (abscissa) would be expressed as 20%. Many technicians do not bother to determine the control time daily but measure the control time in a pool of normal individuals, once for each lot of reagent, and utilize this value throughout the use of that particular lot. In this case, although the error introduced is not important, the expression of prothrombin time as per cent is not really as accurate as a simple reading of the patient's prothrombin time in seconds.

Other side-effects of dicumarol are extreme lassitude, epi-

TYPICAL PROTHROMBIN ACTIVITY CURVES

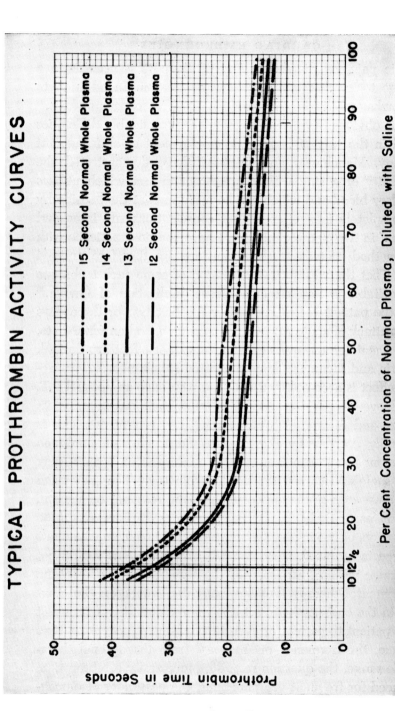

Fig. 5. *Conversion Chart* for typical prothrombin activity curves. The per cent concentration is determined by using as the ordinate point the measured prothrombin time of the patient in seconds. This time is continued horizontally until it intercepts the curve corresponding to the prothrombin time of a normal control. The abscissa is read off from the point where the ordinate intersects the appropriate curve.

gastric pain, or diarrhoea. Any of them may necessitate a change to another anticoagulant preparation. In addition to hemorrhage heparin can produce alopecia or anaphylaxis.[36]

It is obvious from the foregoing that formidable difficulties stand in the way of large-scale employment of anticoagulant therapy. Manchester and Rabkin [37] have demonstrated the feasibility of a single blood prothrombin test which utilizes capillary blood and which can be performed at the bedside by "a completely inexperienced but conscientious and interested person" in two or three minutes. I have had no experience with the method; details of the procedure are therefore omitted here. That the widespread utilization of some such technique is inevitable is implicit in a recent publication of Owren.[38]

If the patient is first seen after the first two or three days of his attack of acute myocardial infarction, and an immediate, then a maintained prolonged anticoagulant effect are desired, heparin and dicumarol may be started simultaneously. An abrupt effect is accomplished with heparin; once an optimal P.T. is achieved heparin is stopped abruptly without tapering its dosage and dicumarol continued for longer term use. This is generally possible by the third or fourth day of combined treatment but it is not an easy procedure since heparin may have some effect upon the prothrombin time. The conversion to the use of a single anticoagulant drug may not be smooth. This is particularly true where large doses of heparin (400 mgms. i.m. or 200 mgms. i.v.) are needed. If such large amounts of heparin are used, blood for P.T. determinations should not be drawn within four hours of the administration of heparin.

Dicumarol therapy thus has many disadvantages: the slowness in the onset of its effect, the unpredictability of its effect from patient to patient or even in the same patient from time to time, the frequency of "escapes" from the optimal therapeutic range, the question regarding uniformity of absorption, the need for frequent venipunctures, the possibility of damaging precious veins and the fastidious nature of the chemical tests themselves. All of these factors have led to dissatisfaction with the drug and to the quest for newer, safer and more effective anticoagulant compounds. Among these have been cyclocumerol (Cumopyron), ethyl biscoumacetate (Tromexan), phenindione (Hedulin, Danilone) and diphenedione (Dipaxin). All of these compounds, excepting Tromexan, have a long induction period. The maintenance of an optimal therapeutic range of prothrombin time is difficult with them. Tromexan works rapidly but control of the prothrombin time with this substance is particularly difficult. Hedulin is subject to the slight but definite risk of inducing agranulocytosis, skin rashes [35] and other sensitivity reactions.[39,40] A new coumarin compound, Coumadin Sodium or Warfarin Sodium has recently come into widespread use and has been the subject of a number of favorable reports.[41-47] My own experience during the past two years has been principally with this drug. It is as rapidly effective as Tromexan but its hypoprothrombinemic effect is more stable and prolonged. Being water-soluble it can also be given by vein; this represents a theoretical advantage, for the use of this drug need not be interrupted in the rare contingency that the patient cannot for a time take the drug by mouth. An optimal range of prothrombin time is generally attained within 36 hours, certainly by 48 hours. There has seemed to me to be less tendency to "escape" with this drug than with dicumarol. I have used it successfully where dicumarol therapy has been clearly ineffective or difficult. I have preferred to administer an initial dose of 50 or 60 mgms., rather than the somewhat larger doses commonly recommended, and to maintain a prolonged prothrombin time by continuous daily administration of the drug. A larger initial dose (up to 75 mgm.) may be given to particularly heavy individuals or smaller initial doses to very light individuals. Smaller doses may be necessary during the period of induction when large amounts of heparin are given at the same time. For those accustomed to dicumarol it must be emphasized that the prothrombin time measured 24 hours after giving the initial dose does not represent its peak effect. As a practical matter, measurement of the 24 hour level may be omitted; if determined at all, it is merely to establish the fact that the prothrombin time is lengthening. The second dose is commonly given at about 48 hours after the initial dose. Depending upon this determination, the following schedule has been recommended as a useful guide to the second dose: [47]

Prothrombin Activity (%)	Dose of Coumadin (mgms.)
10–15	0
15–20	10
20–25	15
25–30	20
30–40	25

As with dicumarol the maintenance dose is then determined by trial and error; it is commonly between 5 and 10 mgms. per day. The administration of the drug in the evening [46] seems to be associated with more uniform absorption and smoother control. The same precautions must be taken in the concomitant administration of heparin and coumadin as are necessary in simultaneous heparin-dicumarol therapy.

Hemorrhage may develop as a complication of anticoagulant therapy for myocardial infarction. This may occur anywhere in the body, even with apparently good laboratory control, but hemorrhage from a peptic ulcer is particularly apt to be disastrous. Attention has been called to the occasional development under these circumstances of hemorrhagic effusion into the pericardium,[48] apparently due to the diapedesis of red cells from the fragile capillaries of the infarcted subepicardial myocardium. Although in many cases this may be harmless, in some it is associated with the development of fatal cardiac tamponade. For this reason it has been recommended that the hypoprothrombinemia be corrected immediately if signs develop of massive pericardial effusion or tamponade, or if a friction rub appears after the first week of the clinical episode, if a friction rub is persistent over a long period of time, or if a friction rub, having appeared during the first week and disappeared, subsequently reappears. If cardiac tamponade develops, a pericardial tap may need to be done. (See page 356.)

Uterine bleeding from anticoagulants is rare. The indication for anticoagulant therapy is unusual in the pre-menopausal woman. Furthermore uterine bleeding is partly controlled by the contraction of the circular smooth muscle surrounding the uterine vessels. This mechanical process is quite independent of the clotting mechanism. However, it must be recognized that menorrhagia or metrorrhagia can be and has been brought about by excessive lowering of the prothrombin time, particularly when the prothrombic activity level falls below 10%.

Although it has been argued by some that the initiation of this form of therapy is just as much an emergency procedure during the incipient or premonitory phase of acute myocardial infarction as it is during well-documented acute infarction, this opinion is not yet generally accepted. Recent studies [49,50] do appear to have confirmed, at least in certain groups and for certain periods, earlier claims [51,52] on the efficacy of long-term anticoagulant prophylaxis against recurrent myocardial infarction. Except to note that hemorrhage is a more frequent complication in this group than in those being treated during an acute episode, this subject need not further concern us here. We may, however, be compelled to treat the complicating emergencies which may, iatrogenic, arise out of its use. Their management is that given when the drugs are used for an acute indication. Patients on constant long-term anticoagulant therapy should be warned about the possibility of dangerous

[77]

hemorrhage in the event of injury and should be on the watch for nosebleed, black and blue marks, black stools or blood in the urine. It would seem wise for such individuals to carry identification cards, similar to those carried by diabetics, stating that they should be given parenteral vitamin K_1 oxide in the event of hemorrhage. They should also carry a supply of this preparation for oral use.

As in the case of the digitalis preparations, it is recommended that one should employ that anticoagulant agent with which he is most familiar. I have had very little experience with Hedulin, none with Dipaxin. It is worth pointing out that a recent large-scale comparison of dicumarol, Warfarin, Hedulin and Dipaxin[53] indicates that the majority of patients can be well controlled with any of these drugs and that none of them appears to have enough advantage over the others to justify recommendation as the prothrombinopenic agent of choice.

During the last few years considerable interest has been awakened in the use of the thrombolytic agents, including streptokinase and streptodornase in the management of arterial and venous thrombosis. An evaluation of this form of therapy in these diseases would be premature at this time.

REFERENCES

(1) Blumgart, H. L., Schlesinger, M. J. and Zoll, P. M.: Angina pectoris, coronary failure and acute myocardial infarction. The rôle of coronary occlusions and collateral circulation. J.A.M.A. 116: 91, 1941.
(2) Master, A. M., Jaffe, H. L., Dack, S. and Grishman, A.: Coronary occlusion, coronary insufficiency and angina pectoris. Am. Ht. J. 27: 803, 1944.
(3) Levine, S. A. and Harvey, W. P.: Temporary relief of anginal pain by carotid sinus stimulation. Tr. A. Am. Physicians 60: 225, 1947.

(4) Sprague, H. B. and White, P. D.: Nitroglycerin collapse
—a potential danger in therapy. Report of three cases.
Med. Clin. No. Am. 16: 895, 1933.

(5) Russek, H. I., Urbach, K. F. and Zohman, B. L.: Paradoxical action of glyceryl trinitrate (nitroglycerin) in
coronary patients. J.A.M.A. 158: 1017, 1955.

(6) Lueth, H. C. and Hanks, T. G.: Unusual reactions of patients with hypertension to glyceryl trinitrate. Arch. Int.
Med. 62: 97, 1938.

(7) Weiss, S., Wilkins, R. W. and Haynes, F. W.: The nature
of circulatory collapse induced by sodium nitrite. J.C.I.
16: 73, 1937.

(8) Wilkins, R. W., Haynes, F. W. and Weiss, S.: The rôle of
the venous system in circulatory collapse induced by sodium nitrite. J.C.I. 16: 85, 1937.

(9) Harrison, T. R. and Finks, R. M.: Glucose deficiency as a
factor in the production of symptoms referable to the
cardiovascular system. Am. Ht. J. 26: 147, 1943.

(10) Halonen, P. I. and Taipale, E.: Angina pectoris as a
symptom of spontaneous hypoglycemia. Cardiologia 20:
243, 1952.

(11) Brooks, H.: Symposium on alcohol: use of alcohol in circulatory defects of old age. M.J. and Rec. 127: 199, 1928.

(12) Stearns, S., Riseman, J. E. F. and Gray, W.: Alcohol in
the treatment of angina pectoris. N.E.J. Med. 234: 578,
1946.

(13) Russek, H. I., Smith, R. H., Baum, W. S., Naegele, C. F.
and Regan, F. D.: Influence of saline, papaverine, nitroglycerin and ethyl alcohol on electrocardiographic
response to standard exercise in coronary disease. Circulation 1: 700, 1950.

(14) Büchner, F.: Die Koronarinsuffizienz, Dresden and Leip-
zig, Theodore Steinkopf, 1939.

(15) Master, A. M., Jaffe, H. L., Field, L. E. and Donoso, E.:

Acute coronary insufficiency: its differential diagnosis and treatment. Ann. Int. Med. 45: 561, 1956.

(16) Graham, D. M., Lyon, T. P., Gofman, J. W., Jones, H. B., Yankley, A., Simonton, J. and White, S.: Blood lipids and human atherosclerosis. II. The influence of heparin upon lipoprotein metabolism. Circulation 4: 666, 1951.

(17) Russek, H. I., Urbach, K. F. and Doerner, A. A.: Effect of heparin in cases of coronary insufficiency. Evaluation by electrocardiographic tests. J.A.M.A. 149: 1008, 1952.

(18) Solandt, D. Y. and Best, C. H.: Heparin and coronary thrombosis in experimental animals. Lancet 2: 130, 1938.

(19) Blumgart, H. L., Schlesinger, M. J. and Zoll, P. M.: Multiple fresh coronary occlusions in patients with antecedent shock. Arch. Int. Med. 68: 181, 1941.

(20) Wexler, J. and Ellis, L. B.: Toxic reactions to the intravenous injection of mercurials. Am. Ht. J. 27: 86, 1944.

(21) Bresnick, E., Woodard, W. K. and Sageman, C. B.: Fatal reactions to intravenous administration of aminophylline. Report of three cases. J.A.M.A. 136: 397, 1948.

(22) Hyman, H. T.: Fatal reactions after aminophylline. J.A.M.A. 136: 895, 1948.

(23) Dolan, L. P.: Allergic death due to intravenous use of diodrast. J.A.M.A. 114: 138, 1940.

(24) Fitz, R.: A case of angina pectoris with cardiac infarct induced by the intravenous injection of sodium tetra-iodo-phenolphthalein and followed by relief of anginoid symptoms. Trans. Assn. Am. Phys. 93: 292, 1928.

(25) Wilcox, H. B., Jr. and Andrus, E. C.: Anaphylaxis in the isolated heart. J. Exper. Med. 67: 169, 1938.

(26) Katz, L. N., Weinstein, W. and Jochim, K.: The coronary vasoconstrictor action of foreign species blood. Am. Ht. J. 15: 452, 1938.

(27) Scherf, D. and Weissberg, J.: Hypertonic glucose solution in angina pectoris. Am. Ht. J. *18*: 411, 1939.

(28) Altschule, M. D. and Gilligan, D. R.: The effects on the cardiovascular system of fluids administered intravenously in man. II. The dynamics of the circulation. J.C.I. *17*: 401, 1938.

(29) Murphy, F. D.: The response of the cardiovascular system to intravenous fluids. J. Urol. *45*: 654, 1941.

(30) Russek, H. I., Regan, F. D. and Naegele, C. F.: One hundred per cent oxygen in the treatment of acute myocardial infarction and severe angina pectoris. J.A.M.A. *144*: 373, 1950.

(31) Proger, S. H. and Ayman, D.: Harmful effects of nitroglycerin with special reference to coronary thrombosis. Am. J. Med. Sci. *184*: 480, 1932.

(32) Wright, I. S., Marple, C. D. and Beck, D. F.: Myocardial Infarction. Its Clinical Manifestations and Treatment with Anticoagulants. A Study of 1031 Cases. Grüne and Stratton, New York, 1954.

(33) Jorpes, J. E.: Heparin in the Treatment of Thrombosis: an account of its Chemistry. Physiology and Application in Medicine. Oxford University Press, London, New York, Toronto, Second Edition, 1946, p. 219.

(34) Tulloch, J. A. and Gilchrist, A. R.: Anticoagulants in the treatment of coronary thrombosis. Brit. Med. J. *2*: 965, 1950.

(35) Breneman, G. M. and Priest, E. M.: Experience with phenylindanedione in the management of acute myocardial infarction. Am. Ht. J. *50*: 129, 1955.

(36) Newcomb, T. F.: Current concepts in therapy. Anticoagulants. N.E.J. Med. *260*: 545, 1959.

(37) Manchester, B. and Rabkin, B.: The control of dicumarol therapy in myocardial infarction by a simple prothrombin test. Circ. *10*: 691, 1954.

(38) Owren, P. A.: Thrombotest. A new method for controlling anticoagulant therapy. Lancet 2: 754, 1959.

(39) Brown, K. W. G. and MacMillan, R. L.: The choice of an anticoagulant. Am. J. Med. Sci. 227: 526, 1954.

(40) Mahous, N. and Vander Veer, J. B.: Severe drug sensitivity reaction to phenindione (phenyldanedione). J.A.M.A. 155: 739, 1954.

(41) Nicholson, J. H. and Leavitt, T., Jr.: Coumadin (Warfarin) Sodium, a new anticoagulant. N.E.J. Med. 255: 491, 1956.

(42) Pollock, B. E.: Clinical experience with Warfarin (Coumadin) Sodium, a new anticoagulant. J.A.M.A. 159: 1094, 1955.

(43) Kerrin, H. F., Guidot, J. and Wilhelm, S. K.: Clinical experience with the anticoagulant Coumadin (Warfarin) Sodium. Angiology, 8: 302, 1957.

(44) Nicholson, J. M.: Clinical experiences with anticoagulants. A comparison of Coumadin (Warfarin) Sodium and Dicumarol (Bishydroxycoumarin). Angiology 8: 456, 1957.

(45) Shapiro, S. and Ciferri, F. E.: Intramuscular administration of the anticoagulant Warfarin (Coumadin) Sodium. J.A.M.A. 165: 1377, 1957.

(46) Fremont, R. E. and Jagendorf, B.: Clinical observations on use of Warfarin (Coumadin) Sodium, a new anticoagulant. J.A.M.A. Ibid. p. 1381.

(47) Porter, R. R., Richardson, D. and Mauck, H. P.: Clinical experiences with the anticoagulant Warfarin Sodium ("Coumadin Sodium"). Virginia Med. Monthly, 85: 465, 1958.

(48) Goldstein, R. and Wolff, L.: Hemorrhagic pericarditis in acute myocardial infarcts treated with bishydroxycoumarin. J.A.M.A. 146: 616, 1951.

(49) Bjerkelund, C. J.: The Effect of Long Term Treatment

with Dicoumarol in Myocardial Infarction. A Controlled Clinical Study. Grüne and Stratton, Inc., New York, London, 1957.

(50) Pickering, G., Arnott, W. M., Biggs, R., Fullerton, H. W., Gilchrist, A. R., Hunter, R. B., Reid, D. D., Wood, P., Wright, J. H. and Douglas, A. S.: An assessment of long-term anticoagulant administration after cardiac infarction. Report of the working party on anticoagulant therapy in coronary thrombosis to the Medical Research Council. Brit. M.J. *1*: 5125, 1959.

(51) Nichol, E. S. and Fassett, E. W.: An attempt to forestall acute coronary thrombosis. Preliminary note on the continuous use of dicumarol. South Med. J. *40*: 631, 1947.

(52) Nichol, E. S., Keyes, J. N., Borg, J. F., Coogan, T. J., Boehrer, J. J., Mullins, W. L., Scott, T., Page, R., Griffith, G. C. and Massie, E.: Long-term anticoagulant therapy in coronary atherosclerosis. Am. Ht. J. *55*: 142, 1958.

(53) Rodman, T., Ryan, C. S., Pastor, B. H. and Hollendonner, W. J. with the technical assistance of Harrison, E.: A comparative study of four prothrombinopenic anticoagulant drugs. II. Clinical study. Am. J. Med. *27*: 415, 1959.

4

UNUSUAL AND NON-CARDIAC

CAUSES OF CHEST PAIN

Dissecting Aneurysm of the Aorta

Acute Mediastinal Emphysema

Nerve Root Pain

Rupture of the Esophagus

Acute Pericarditis

Chest Wall Pain

Anterior Chest Wall Syndrome

Precordial Catch

Hiatus Hernia and Peptic Esophagitis

Spontaneous Pneumothorax

CHAPTER

4

UNUSUAL AND NON-CARDIAC

CAUSES OF CHEST PAIN

There is a common tendency, among laymen and physicians alike, to attribute all chest pain to heart disease.
But there is a considerable catalogue of extra-cardiac disorders
capable of inducing this symptom. To a greater or lesser extent
these can simulate the chest pain of acute myocardial infarction. This list includes: dissecting aneurysm of the aorta; acute
pleurisy (interlobar or diaphragmatic); acute pneumothorax;
pulmonary infarction or acute cor pulmonale; acute pneumonia; acute pericarditis; impending diabetic coma; acute mediastinal emphysema; acute gall bladder disease; erosion and
perforation of the esophagus; penetrating peptic ulcer; acute
pancreatitis; diaphragmatic hernia; herpes zoster; arthritis of
the spine; carcinoma of the lung; and syphilitic aneurysm
of the aorta. The list is legion. It would be worth-while, however, to dwell at some length upon a few of these conditions.
Some of them, being rare, are not familiar to most physicians.
Some, like dissecting aneurysm, are truly vascular emergencies.
Others, like acute mediastinal emphysema or ruptured esophagus, are not vascular emergencies at all, but may simulate
them.

DISSECTING ANEURYSM OF THE AORTA

An ante-mortem diagnosis of dissecting aneurysm of the aorta is possible in perhaps 25 to 35% of cases. The pain may resemble that of acute myocardial infarction. It is generally sudden in onset, extreme in intensity and described variously as tearing, knife-like, crushing, excruciating, unbearable or throbbing and is frequently associated with the development of shock.[1] The pain may begin in the chest, in the back, in the neck, in the back of the throat or in the epigastrium. Much more important than the initial site of the pain is its tendency to change location. After a shorter or longer period following the onset of the attack, the pain tends to become less intense in the chest or epigastrium and now manifests itself between the shoulder blades or in the small of the back or down the legs. Generally the pain does not radiate down the arms unless the brachial circulation is compromised.[2] Another extremely helpful point in the diagnosis of dissecting aneurysm is the fact that it develops almost exclusively in individuals who have been or are hypertensive. The exception to this rule is the peculiar predilection to aortic dissection during pregnancy in women with coarctation of the aorta. There is a pronounced tendency in patients with dissecting aneurysm for the blood pressure to remain elevated even during the acute clinical episode. Of course, if the patient loses a large amount of blood or goes into shock for other reasons, his blood pressure will fall. In dissecting aneurysm, however, hypotension is much less common than in acute myocardial infarction. Gallop rhythm and cardiac arrhythmias, so common during coronary thrombosis, are not observed in dissecting aneurysm. Logue's sign [3] which consists of a pulsation in either sternoclavicular joint may be extremely helpful in this diagnosis.

The remainder of the symptomatology of dissecting aneurysm

may be extremely varied [1] and dependent upon which of the branches of the thoracic and abdominal portions of the aorta is, or are, involved. Faintness or fainting, which occasionally follows soon after the onset of the pain, may be related to compression of the innominate or the left common carotid artery. Weiss [2] suggested that these symptoms might be related to irritation of the receptors which are located in the arch of the aorta. Giddiness, blurring of vision, even blindness, and paralyses may result from obstruction of one of these vessels. Encroachment upon the origin of the left subclavian artery may be signaled by decrease or disappearance of the left radial pulse previously known to be present. Occlusion of the intercostal arteries may be manifested by symmetrical paraplegias, the result of local ischemia of the spinal cord. Involvement of the mesenteric arteries can result in abdominal pain from mesenteric thrombosis. At times, the palpating hand may detect the presence and progressive enlargement of a tender, pulsating mass in the abdomen. This may even be the site of a thrill or murmur. Extension of the process to the aortic bifurcation may be manifested by loss of the femoral pulsations. When this diagnosis is suspected, it is extremely important therefore to conduct careful, systematic and repeated examinations of the palpability of all accessible pulsations. It is essential moreover that any observed inequality between the two sides be recorded immediately—before the observation is forgotten.

The process may dissect its way proximally, involve the orifices of the coronary arteries and induce coronary insufficiency or acute myocardial infarction. At times, this complication may be the result not of throttling of the orifices of the coronary arteries but of massive hemorrhage and shock. The electrocardiogram may then show, over and above the left ventricular hypertrophy which is an almost invariable antecedent of this condition, evidence of coronary insufficiency or of myocardial infarction. Thus in rare cases the question may be not whether there is dissecting aneurysm *or* myocardial infarction, but whether there is dissecting aneurysm *and* myocardial infarction. Another consequence of proximal dissection is a narrowing of the aortic lumen just above the aortic valve ring. This distorts the aortic valve leaflets out of their normally apposing relationship. There is some difference of opinion on how this is brought about. Some attribute it to a dilatation of the aortic ring. This produces a diastolic murmur which is audible over the entire precordium but which is maximal in intensity in the aortic valve area. In fact the detection of such a murmur not previously present, in a hypertensive patient with severe chest or abdominal pain, is almost diagnostic of dissecting aneurysm of the aorta. At times, this heralds the imminence of pericardial bleeding. Cardiac tamponade may be slow but is generally rapid in development. If there is a slow ooze of blood into the pericardium, a pericardial friction rub may be heard and the electrocardiogram may show evidence of pericarditis. This is probably the effect of deposition of fibrin on the epicardial surface from the pericardial blood. Thus in dissecting aneurysm the electrocardiogram may show evidence of left ventricular hypertrophy, of myocardial ischemia or infarction, or of pericarditis. Rapid tamponade may be indicated by an abrupt deterioration in the condition of the patient, by enlargement of the area of cardiac dullness, by disappearance of the apex impulse, by a decreased intensity or absence of the heart sounds, by a fall in blood pressure, by an increase in venous pressure, by tachypnea and by tachycardia. Severe cardiac embarrassment can result from the rapid entrance of relatively small amounts of blood into the pericardial sac. Fatal tamponade may in fact be produced by as little as 200 to 500 cc. On the other hand, when bleeding is slow, relatively large amounts of blood are tolerated with little embarrassment.

The X-ray examination offers some limited assistance in the

diagnosis of dissecting aneurysm. A decision must be made whether the condition of the patient justifies his being brought to the X-Ray department for films. If this is considered inadvisable, bedside portable films should be taken but these are generally not so satisfactory. At times, dissection of the thoracic or abdominal aorta may be demonstrated by a widening of the aortic shadow in the corresponding region (Fig. 6). Enlargement of the cardiac contour is also seen when a slow leak into the pericardium produces a large effusion, though it must be differentiated from the cardiac shadow of congestive heart failure. In rapidly developing tamponade enlargement of cardiac size may not occur. Fluoroscopy may show absence of cardiac pulsation. The diagnosis and management of pericardial tamponade is discussed further on pages 353–357.

Secondary rupture is the principal cause of death. This occurs into the pericardium in about 75% of cases,[4] into the left pleural space in 20% and into the mediastinum in the remaining 5% or so. In a small, uncertain percentage of cases the patient may survive his dissection by months or years.[5] This appears to be related in some cases to re-entrance of the dissection into the main aortic lumen. The patient may then have a double-barreled aorta consisting of a tube within a tube.

Until recently, treatment has been one of hopeful waiting, analgesia, sedation and maximal rest in bed for 6 to 8 weeks.[4] Anticoagulants, of course, are withheld. Transfusions are necessary if there is severe loss of blood. Pericardial paracentesis is futile except as an immediate measure since blood re-accumulates from the unaffected bleeding area. Surgical efforts to ligate the site of rupture or wrapping of the aorta with cellophane or gelfoam have been tried but have been ineffective. More recently some courageous surgeons have felt that the inexorable progress of this catastrophe might be halted by deliberately re-establishing a communication between the distal part of the dissection and the original aortic lumen.[6] I know of

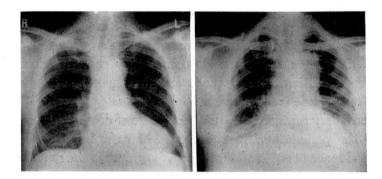

Fig. 6. *Increasing Aortic Shadow in Dissecting Aneurysm of the Aorta.* A 56-year-old hypertensive baseball fan developed severe pain in the chest and epigastrium, radiating to the small of the back during a scoring spree. Initial chest film (left) showed large left ventricle, an unremarkable aorta. Pain continued and next day spread down right arm. Subsequent film (right) showed widening of mediastinum with fuzziness of aorta. At P.M. dissection extended from aortic arch to iliac arteries with secondary rupture of arch near origin of left subclavian artery.

one or two cases in which this has been accomplished successfully. Excisional therapy with graft replacement, as practiced
by DeBakey,[6] has been even more encouraging. The mortality
rate attending these procedures will necessarily be high but in
dealing with such a deadly process as dissecting aneurysm they
are probably worth the candle.

ACUTE MEDIASTINAL EMPHYSEMA

Another cause of chest pain is the entrance of air into the
mediastinal structures. The increased pressure in the mediastinum is presumably responsible for the chest pain. There is good
evidence that the cause of this condition is the rupture of certain of the pulmonary alveoli.[7] The air which thus escapes from
the air sacs generally dissects its way proximally along the
bronchi to the mediastinum. An abruptly increased intrathoracic pressure, particulary against a closed glottis, during a
paroxysm of coughing is commonly responsible. In this way
mediastinal emphysema may complicate many conditions
such as the laryngeal obstruction of diphtheria or pertussis, the
bronchospasm of asthma, the act of parturition, heavy lifting or
violent straining as at stool, or other conditions in which the
intrathoracic pressure is increased and the glottis closed.[7] It
occasionally develops in newborn infants after efforts at resuscitation. In adults it has on occasion appeared in association
with intratracheal insufflation, intratracheal anaesthesia, glass
blowing or playing wind instruments. It has been described as
a complication of influenza, pneumonia or tuberculosis. But, as
pointed out by Hamman,[8,9] it may develop occasionally without
obvious antecedent strain. The use of the term "spontaneous"
mediastinal emphysema for such cases has been criticised by
Aisner and Franco.[10] These authors point out that the condition
may be slow in developing and that a precipitating factor which
was operative several days previously might have been over-

looked or have escaped detection since they were not mentioned by the patient or inquired into by the physician. Mediastinal emphysema also develops secondarily to fractured ribs, blast injuries, other forms of chest trauma, caisson disease, rupture of the esophagus and the like.[10] In general, mediastinal emphysema affects a younger age population than that inclined to coronary disease.

If the pressure of air in the mediastinum becomes sufficiently increased the venous return will be impeded, leading to a fall in cardiac output similar to that seen in pericardial tamponade. At this time the trapped air may threaten the life of the patient and constitute an acute medical emergency. The air may escape from the mediastinum into the neck and thence beneath the skin of the chest, axillae, abdomen and genitalia. Or it may escape into either pleural space (pneumothorax), into the pericardium (pneumopericardium) or into the retroperitoneal space (retropneumoperitoneum) and thence into the abdominal cavity (pneumoperitoneum). No matter what the route of egress, the decrease of mediastinal pressure thus affected is followed by complete or partial relief of the patient's chest pain.

Chest pain is the most common symptom of mediastinal emphysema. This is generally abrupt in onset and located beneath the abdomen, over the pericardium, in the left axilla or between the scapulae. Radiation to the neck, to the left shoulder and arm or to the back, is often described. The intensity of the discomfort varies from little more than a sense of oppression or constriction, to a severe, sharp, stabbing, knife-like or squeezing pain.[11] It may therefore resemble the pain of angina pectoris or myocardial infarction. The younger age of most patients whose chest pain is due to mediastinal emphysema generally diverts the attention of the physician from coronary artery disease and alerts his interest in this possibility. The duration varies from minutes to days. At times the pain is made worse when the patient lies on his left side and is relieved by sitting up. Some patients feel a crackling sensation in the chest at the same time, or complain of pain on swallowing or on turning the head. At times the chest pain is associated with dyspnea, cyanosis, anxiety, perspiration or palpitation.

The detection of fine crackling or crepitant râles over the precordium, synchronous with the heart beat, is diagnostic of mediastinal emphysema. These are heard in systole alone or in both systole and diastole; in the latter instance they are louder in systole. In addition to these crepitations a loud popping sound may be heard, which may long outlast the crepitations. Commonly the patient, and occasionally with great delight, can maneuver himself into a certain position in which he can hear and feel and demonstrate his own sounds. Not all observers describe these sounds in this way; depending upon the ingenuity and imagination of the author, a veritable thesaurus of alternative designations has been offered. They have been described as crackling, bubbling, crunching, rattling, grinding or snapping, or resembling the crinkling of a newspaper or the sound of walking in crisp dry snow on a quiet day.[11] In contrast to the more continuous rubbing quality of a pericardial friction rub these sounds are more discrete, interrupted and consonating. A second physical sign of mediastinal emphysema is a hyper-resonant or tympanitic percussion note over the precordium. Subcutaneous emphysema in the neck, axillae, chest or abdominal wall or in the scrotum and signs of pneumothorax or pneumoperitoneum should be sought. With the exception to be noted below the patient shows very little if any constitutional reaction in spite of his chest pain. The "vital signs" —temperature, heart rate, respiratory rate and blood pressure— remain normal. There is no shock. Leucocytosis, elevation of the sedimentation rate and important electrocardiographic changes are absent.

Careful examination with roentgenograms and fluoroscopy

may disclose the presence of air in the mediastinum. In the lateral view in particular a collection of air is often seen between the front of the heart and the inside of the sternum. In the anteroposterior view a band of markedly increased radiotranslucency is seen parallel to the left cardiac border. This delineates air between the parietal pericardium and adjacent parietal pleura. The failure to follow faithfully the cardiac silhouette and absence of fluid level distinguishes this from a pneumopericardium.

Treatment. The prime fear or conviction of the patient and his associates will generally be that he is suffering a heart attack. He must be assured at once that this is not so and that his condition is not serious. Generally nothing more is necessary than symptomatic treatment of his pain and provision of a period of rest in bed or chair adequate to permit resorption of air from the mediastinal tissues. Since there is a slight tendency to recurrence, particularly in the event of persistence or recurrence of the conditions which brought about his original attack, a period of follow-up observation is advisable.

In a few exceptional cases, however, when increasing amounts of air build up in the mediastinum and there is no possibility of its spontaneous escape, the symptoms of tamponade may develop with increasing pain, dyspnea, cyanosis, suffocation, suffusion of face and neck, tachycardia, hypotension, shock and, if unrelieved, death. In this emergency situation release of the pent-up mediastinal air should be done promptly through a supraclavicular or thyroidectomy incision. This is preferable to blind needling which can injure the great veins. Nevertheless there are undoubtedly situations of such compelling emergency that this risk will have to be accepted and venting of air performed through a needle. Where a tension pneumothorax has complicated the mediastinal emphysema, the aspiration of air from the pleura and the provision of a water-seal drain may indirectly relieve the mediastinal pressure. Adequate analgesia and sedation are mandatory. Oxygen therapy should be given but this should never be of the positive-pressure variety.[12]

NERVE ROOT PAIN

Certain pathological processes in or about the nerve roots of the cervical or upper thoracic spine may produce chest pain.[13,14] Local injury, particularly whip-lash injuries, fracture of a posterior facet or of a vertebral arch, postural and occupational strains and subluxations, osteoarthritis, root sleeve fibrosis or, more rarely, tumor or shingles, are often causes of chest pain. Compression of nerve roots by a ruptured disc is uncommon in the cervical spine.[14] These conditions may involve the nerve roots in their course within the spinal canal or as they pass through the intervertebral foramina. When the dorsal root is involved, the pain may be lancinating and radiate widely; when the ventral root is affected, the pain may be deep, dull, boring or aching. It is likely to be more prolonged and associated with soreness in the muscle and skin and resemble the pressing, crushing and vise-like discomfort ordinarily associated with coronary artery disease. It is commonly related to certain positions of the head and neck or to damp weather; at other times a story of such a relationship can be ferreted out only with great difficulty. It may be precipitated or aggravated by coughing, deep breathing, laughing, sneezing or straining at stool. It occurs at times on walking but, unlike the pain of angina pectoris, it appears to be related more to a painful jarring of the spine produced by each step; it does not cease promptly on stopping and, in fact it may be due to an unconscious straightening out of the spine when the patient stops. Often the patient is capable of more exertion without developing pain. It is apt to be worse after prolonged recumbency. The pain is commonly associated with stiffness of muscles, with numbness and tingling in the skin and with parasternal tenderness. It is generally felt in the neck and shoulders but it may spread beneath the clavicles, to the axilla or even the precordium. Primary pain in, or radiation to, the substernal region has been described from root irritation [13] but this has been extremely rare in my experience. In fact, the diagnostic problem has not been so much whether a patient presents *either* coronary *or*, nerve root pain but whether he has *both* coronary *and* nerve root pain.

On examination the physician will find that the head cannot be turned in its entire 180 degree range. Percussion over, or direct or oblique pressure upon, individual spinous or transverse processes of the cervical or upper thoracic vertebrae will not only disclose sharply localized tenderness but it may also duplicate the radiation of the spontaneous pain of which the patient complains. On roentgen examination one should look for narrowing of the intervertebral spaces in the antero-posterior projection and narrowing of the intervertebral foramina in the oblique views. Bony spurs constitute another important lead to the correct diagnosis. Skin tenderness, muscle spasm and weakness or paresis of muscles are other commonly associated findings. Furthermore traction applied manually or with a special apparatus including sling, pulley and weights, may afford striking relief of the pain. According to Jackson [14] the injection of local anaesthetic into painful muscles of cervical root irritation characteristically does two things. First it reproduces the radicular pattern of pain momentarily; then it affords dramatic relief of this pain for intervals that vary from days to weeks or even months.

Treatment can often be simple and symptomatic but occasionally more elaborate orthopedic measures are necessary. Heat, applied as hot moist packs or diathermy and accompanied by gentle massage, are helpful. The injection in a stellate manner of ½% procaine solution or of lipocaine hydrochloride

(Xylocaine) into the area of maximal tenderness is effective as a diagnostic as well as therapeutic measure. Continuous or intermittent traction, immobilization of the spine with a shoulder brace or Thomas collar or the use at night of a cervical contour pillow should be considered. If these measures are ineffective, paravertebral block or local infiltration of the scalenus anticus muscle with procaine should be tried. In the rare case in which a protruded cervical disc is recognized and conservative therapy is ineffectual, surgery may be necessary.

RUPTURE OF THE ESOPHAGUS

Severe vomiting or retching, particularly after the ingestion of large amounts of food and drink can induce linear tears in the lower esophagus just above the cardio-esophageal junction. These perforations may extend only into the mediastinum but more commonly enter the left pleural space. The clinical picture is one of the most dramatic and compelling in all of medicine. There is an abrupt development of tachycardia, hypotension and excruciating, tearing pain in the substernal region and in the left side of the chest, associated with severe dyspnea, prostration, splinting of the left side of the chest and grunting respiration.[15] That such rupture occurs at all has been ascribed to pre-existent weakness of the esophageal mucosa. The overwhelming majority of patients succumbing to this catastrophe have been chronic alcoholics. This has been ascribed to long-standing weakness of the mucosa from alcoholic gastritis or esophagitis. In some patients linear tears develop not in the esophagus but in the gastric mucosa near the cardio-esophageal junction.[16] These produce severe hemorrhage but not rupture.

Rupture of the esophagus is followed by the rapid development of pleural effusion, mediastinitis and emphysema of the mediastinum and uncommonly of the subcutaneous tissues. Because of pleural soiling there generally develops a severe hemo-pyo-pneumothorax, pleuritis and pneumonitis. Symptoms of tamponade may develop because of mechanical compression of the vascular structures in the mediastinum.

The X-ray may be of considerable help in the diagnosis of rupture of the esophagus. It may show broadening of the mediastinal shadow and a left pneumothorax with pleural effusion. The latter finding is diagnostic. Air may be seen in the tissues especially at the root of the neck. The detection of air under the diaphragm would be evidence against perforated esophagus and favors a ruptured peptic ulcer. The finding of subcutaneous emphysema in a patient who develops severe pain in the lower chest or upper abdomen, though uncommon, is likewise diagnostic of this condition.[17] If a chest tap is done, the aspirated fluid should be cultured and titrated for free acid. Swallowed lipiodol demonstrated by roentgen ray in the pleural cavity or methylene blue recovered by paracentesis establishes the diagnosis. It must be emphasized that here again the diagnosis has to be thought of to be made.

Until recently this condition was invariably fatal. Only since immediate surgery for repair of the esophageal rent has been employed have any of these patients been saved. A prompt left thoracotomy is the treatment of choice. The esophagus must be exposed and the defect located and sutured. A tube drain is led from the site of repair through a separate stab incision low down on the back of the chest and connected to a water seal. The pleura should be cultured and cleansed, penicillin instilled and the lung re-expanded. The patient must be vigorously supported with blood and plasma and explored in spite of shock. The case described in Fig. 7 was seen at a time when surgery was not considered for this condition. In the light of more recent experience this patient need not have died.

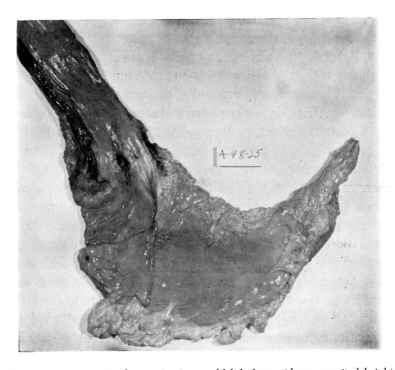

Fig. 7. *Rupture of Esophagus.* A 76-year-old bibulous widower vomited bright red blood while on a drinking bout, developing excruciating epigastric pain which moved to left side of chest, left scapula and back. Heart and abdomen negative. Base of left lung dull on percussion and breath sounds distant. Peripheral pulses equal and synchronous. B.P. 170/80, both arms. Electrocardiogram normal. WBC 13,700. Chest film showed fluid at left base and above this a rounded area of increased translucency with fluid level. Temperature rose to 105.8, heart rate to 140 and respirations to 40. Patient then went into collapse and died 14 hours after admission. P.M.: Elliptical rupture 2 cms. in length, 0.7 cm. in breadth, about 0.5 cm. above cardio-esophageal junction. Probe passed into defect through mediastinum and into left pleural cavity which contained 2000 c.c. of dirty dark fluid. Left lung collapsed. No mediastinal emphysema, liver disease or varices.

[101]

ACUTE PERICARDITIS

The pain of acute benign ("viral" or non-suppurative) pericarditis may at times resemble that of acute myocardial infarction, but it is generally not so severe. It is likely to come on in company with or in the wake of an acute upper respiratory infection. The location is precordial or parasternal and it often radiates to the neck, back or arms and sometimes to the back of the throat. The pain may be pleuritic, but more characteristically it is an ache or deep substernal soreness which is accentuated by inspiration. It may be induced or aggravated by changes in posture such as twisting, turning or bending the chest. In consequence some patients assume an immobile attitude generally bending forward slightly with rapid panting respirations, an unconscious response designed to avoid the postural and pleuritic components of the pain. Dyspnea is almost invariably present and there is occasionally some discomfort in the liver region. A flat percussion note over the lower half, or two-thirds, of the sternum is an extremely helpful sign pointing to significant pericardial effusion.[19] A pericardial friction rub may be heard very early in the course of acute benign pericarditis whereas it generally appears after a number of days in acute myocardial infarction.

The electrocardiogram offers considerable help in this diagnosis. The RS-T shifts recorded in pericarditis rarely attain the degree of elevation that is observed in some cases of acute myocardial infarction. In the first day or two these shifts can, in fact, be distinguished only with great difficulty from similar shifts which may be recorded as a perfectly normal variation in some individuals. A decision between these two possibilities is generally possible from an appraisal of the clinical situation and from serial observations of the electrocardiogram. The earliest change consists of an elevation of the RS-T segment by one or two millimeters. The area over which this change is seen is

somewhat variable but since the process is inclined to dissemi-
nate itself over the entire epicardial surface it is generally seen
in most of the precordial leads and in many of the limb leads.
Early in the acute episode the T wave may remain upright or
even be fairly tall and peaked but generally, in the course of
two or three days the T waves flatten out and, as the RS-T
segments return to the isoelectric line, the T waves become
smartly inverted. These changes proceed much more rapidly
than do similar RS-T and T wave changes in the course of
acute myocardial infarction. Furthermore pronounced "reciprocal" changes like those seen in acute myocardial infarction
are not observed in pericarditis. One may, however, see slight
depression of the RS-T segments in leads aVR, and V_1 or
V_1 and V_2 since these leads may face the endocardial aspect
of the pericardial "current of injury." Pericarditis, moreover,
does not induce changes in the QRS complex. The brisk T wave
inversions may last from one to six or more weeks, then gradually become isoelectric, and finally normally upright. Eventually
a normal looking electrocardiogram is resumed.

Roentgen-ray examination may show enlargement of the
cardiac shadow or fluid at the left lung base. The white count
and sedimentation rate are elevated and the cold agglutination
test positive. This is more impressive if there is a rise in titer but
an initial reaction in 1:40 dilution may be significant.

Only rarely does acute pericarditis become an acute emergency. There are some few patients in whom cardiac tamponade
may develop. This subject is more fully discussed on page 353.
In pericarditis the accumulation of fluid is slow and therefore
the volume of fluid in the pericardial sac may be large. A
pericardial paracentesis may be life saving. If there is good
evidence for tamponade but the amount of effusion seems
small, discretion would indicate that the tap be done by a
surgeon who can actually cut down on the pericardium and
enter it under direct visualization. This eliminates the risk of

entering auricular wall or coronary artery. The operative removal of a disc of pericardial tissue offers the further advantages of yielding biopsy material, frequently permitting a precise pathologic diagnosis, and of providing drainage of effusions from pericardium to adjacent pleura and thence through an intercostal catheter connected to a water-sealed suction apparatus.[20]

Another rare but real emergency is presented by the patient who develops constrictive pericarditis early in the course of his acute pericarditis. Traumatic hemopericardium may lead to early eschar formation and pericardial constriction; this may also follow if inflammatory pericardial fluid is hemorrhagic.[21]

CHEST WALL PAIN

Tietze's Syndrome Another cause of chest pain is a costochondral syndrome described by Tietze.[22] This is a benign, non-infectious and non-suppurative inflammation of obscure pathology and etiology involving one or, uncommonly, more than one, of the costochondral junctions, generally of the second rib, occasionally of other ribs and rarely of the sterno-clavicular junction.[23] The patient, generally a young or middle-aged individual, complains of pain, soreness or tightness in the anterior part of the chest. At times this pain radiates into the neck, shoulder or arm. It is aggravated by sneezing, coughing or bending.[24] Its relation is to movement of the chest wall, not to activity as such. It may be worse on lying down. At times it has followed severe intractable coughing. It is frequently preceded by, or accompanied by, a respiratory infection. Occasionally it seems to be related to damp weather, anxiety, fatigue or poor posture. Examination shows tenderness in the involved costochondral junction or junctions. This may be associated with a bulbous or fusiform swelling of this structure. Compression of the rib cage in the neighborhood induces pain identical with that of which the patient complains. The tenderness is not intercostal in distribution.[25] On being reassured that this is not angina pectoris or cancer of the breast, the patient may no longer note this symptom or he may overlook it. But the course is quite variable and may be prolonged—to months or even years. Treatment consists of firm reassurance that this is a benign condition, the local application of heat, the use of aspirin or local infiltration with procaine. The relief afforded by the latter may long outlast any effect that can be attributed to its purely local analgesic properties. Deep X-ray therapy and oral steroid therapy have also been used.

Anterior Chest Wall Syndrome This is a painful affliction of the anterior chest wall which is said to differ from Tietze's syndrome in that it is located below the level of the second rib and in that there is no swelling of the costochondral junctions. Whether such a distinction is justifiable seems questionable. This condition apparently occurs more frequently in patients who have suffered a coronary occlusion in the recent or remote past. The pain is unrelated to exertion or food, is unrelieved by nitroglycerin, does not radiate and is unassociated with systemic or vasomotor manifestations. It is generally a continuous sort of pain lasting hours and subsiding gradually; it is subject to acute exacerbations which are commonly induced by certain positions of the body or movements of the trunk. Tenderness is diffuse and exquisite and generally located over bones and cartilages in the sternochondral regions or over the cardiac apex. Pain is elicited by pressure on any part of the chest. Especially in individuals with known previous coronary artery disease it may be confused with coronary insufficiency or myocardial infarction and lead to unnecessary invalidism, neurosis or narcotic addiction. The patient with this condition should be reassured that this pain is not due to heart disease and, unless he presents definite evidence of active heart disease, he should be urged to become more active. In some cases this may be all that is necessary. In other patients corticotropin or cortisone may be used in a dose of 100 to 150 mgms. per day for two days, tapering the dose down to 25 mgms. by the end of the first week or ten days. Cortisone may be continued after ACTH is discontinued. If pain continues despite steroids, X-ray therapy may be given for a few days. Procaine infiltration may be especially helpful in demonstrating to the patient the local nature of his pain.

"Precordial Catch" In this condition the patient, generally a person less than 35 years old and of light or medium build, suddenly feels a sharp or knifelike pain in the region of the cardiac apex.[27] The pain returns every time a deep breath is taken so that the patient avoids deep breathing and tends to maintain his chest in the position of expiration or semi-inspiration. The pain does not radiate. It may occur at rest or during mild activity and has been associated with a slouched position. The patient may find that, if he forces himself to take a deep breath, the pain disappears, to be replaced perhaps by a mild ache or discomfort. On examination there is no tenderness or hyperalgesia at the site of pain, no nodules or deformity. The patient should be reassured that his pain is not due to heart disease. If his posture is poor, this should be corrected. Otherwise no treatment is called for.

HIATUS HERNIA AND PEPTIC ESOPHAGITIS

Hiatus hernia can induce a discouragingly variable clinical picture. About 14% of patients with symptomatic hiatus hernia are said[28] to experience a sudden dramatic onset of their symptoms. Such acute symptoms are just about as frequent as the classical hiatus hernia symptom complex of epigastric or substernal burning pain initiated or aggravated by recumbency and relieved by the assumption of the upright posture.

In 7% of cases the subjective symptoms are reported to mimic those of coronary insufficiency or myocardial infarction.[28] In my own experience such confusion has been uncommon; much more often than not the demonstration of a hiatus hernia has served as little more than a snare and a delusion. The point of view of various authorities on the subject seems to vary with their particular interest and their location along the diagnostic-therapeutic production line. The difficulty in diagnosis is compounded by the ubiquity of demonstrable but innocent hiatus hernia and the frequency of associated disease, generally in the abdomen, occasionally in the coronary arteries. If hernia is demonstrated by X-ray or esophagoscopy and measures commonly effective in heart disease have failed to relieve the symptoms, the patient should be treated for hiatus hernia, even if the diagnosis of coronary heart disease is indubitable. Treatment includes a low-calory ulcer-type diet with frequent small meals, alkalis, belladonna or propantheline bromide (Pro-Banthine), assumption of the upright position after meals and elevation of the head of the bed at night. Surgery should be considered for hiatus hernia when there is a previous history of ulceration, stricture or intractable esophagitis, when there is a large hernia presenting the hazard of strangulation, when a thorough-going program of medical therapy has been ineffective or when a medical regimen would be so difficult, complicated or inconvenient that it is unlikely that it would be followed.

Peptic esophagitis is an inflammatory condition of the lower esophagus, said to be due to reflux of acid gastric contents into the lower esophagus, and commonly associated with hiatal hernia, short esophagus, peptic ulcer or with diseases associated with frequent attacks of vomiting.[29] The patient complains of substernal pain made worse by lying down, stooping or bending, of heartburn, sour eructations and dysphagia. The diagnosis is made by esophagoscopy. In my experience even the most expert esophagoscopic and roentgenologic examination can miss carcinoma as the background cause. Ulceration may complicate this condition and lead to minor oozing or severe hemorrhage and acute or chronic anemia of moderate or severe degree. Perforation is a rare complication.

The symptoms of peptic esophagitis are impressively relieved by antacid and ulcer therapy, preferably in combination with vagolytic agents such as tincture of belladonna, atropine, Banthine or Probanthine. The patient should sleep with the head of his bed elevated. Some recommend that bouginage be employed as a prophylaxis against stricture. In symptomatic cases repair of a demonstrated hiatus hernia will relieve the esophagitis and prevent the serious complication of stricture formation. In others emergency surgery will be necessary because of perforation.

SPONTANEOUS PNEUMOTHORAX

Spontaneous pneumothorax characteristically induces pain, tightness or discomfort in the chest and dyspnea. Examination shows decreased breath sounds and decreased tactile fremitus. A distracted or ritual examination can easily miss these findings or the hyperresonance characterizing moderate degree of pneumothorax. As with so many conditions, the most important requisite to the diagnosis is to think of it. X-ray examination should be done if this diagnosis is suspected since small pneumothoraces are often associated with few findings on physical examination. Treatment should be conservative or symptomatic. Re-expansion in these cases may require from a few days to several weeks. Catheter intubation with water-seal suction is employed to accelerate this process if evidence of tension pneumothorax, bleeding, effusion, hemothorax or simultaneous collapse of the other lung is detected. With a large or slowly absorbing pneumothorax it is preferable to re-expand the lung by inserting two needles at different points on the affected side of the chest, one for inflow, the other for outflow, and washing ten liters of oxygen through the pleural cavity in this way. This displaces the inert nitrogen of the pneumothorax with rapidly absorbable oxygen.

Pulmonary embolism or infarction may likewise produce chest pain. This is considered at length in the succeeding chapter.

REFERENCES

(1) Baer, S.: Varied manifestations of dissecting aneurysm of the aorta. J.A.M.A. *161*: 689, 1956.

(2) Weiss, S.: The clinical course of spontaneous dissecting aneurysm of the aorta. Med. Clin. No. Am. Boston number. January 1935. p. 1117.

(3) Logue, R B. and Sikes, C.: A new sign in dissecting aneurysm of aorta. Pulsation of a sternoclavicular joint. J.A.M.A. *148*: 1209, 1952.

(4) Reich, N. E.: Diseases of the Aorta. Diagnosis and Treatment. The MacMillan Company, New York. 1949, p. 130.

(5) Prior, J. T., Buran, R. T. and Perl, T.: Chronic (healed) dissecting aneurysms. J. Thoracic Surg. 33: 213, 1957.

(6) DeBakey, M. E. and Creech, O., Jr.: Surgical treatment of dissecting aneurysm. J.A.M.A. *162*: 1654, 1956.

(7) Macklin, M. T. and Macklin, C. C.: Malignant interstitial emphysema of the lungs and mediastinum as an important occult complication in many respiratory diseases and other conditions: An interpretation of the clinical literature in the light of laboratory experiment. Medicine *23*: 281, 1944.

(8) Hamman, L.: Spontaneous mediastinal emphysema. J. H. H. Bull. *64*: 1, 1939.

(9) Hamman, L.: Mediastinal emphysema. J.A.M.A. *128*: 1, 1945.

(10) Aisner, M. and Franco, J. E.: Medical progress. Mediastinal emphysema. N.E.J. Med. *241*: 818, 1949.

(11) Towbin, M. N.: Mediastinal emphysema occurring with therapeutic pneumoperitoneum: report of 10 cases. Ann. Int. Med. *35*: 555, 1951.

(12) Gaudrault, G. L. and Chalmers, D. M.: Emergency treatment of traumatic emphysema of the mediastinum. N.E.J. Med. *224*: 940, 1941.

(13) Davis, D.: Radicular Syndrome with Emphasis on Chest Pain Simulating Coronary Disease. Year Book Publishers, Inc., Chicago, 1957.

(14) Jackson, R.: The Cervical Syndrome. Charles C. Thomas, Springfield, 1956, p. 37.

(15) Beal, J. M., Jr.: Spontaneous rupture of the esophagus. Ann. Surg. *129*: 512, 1949.

(16) Mallory, G. K. and Weiss, S.: Hemorrhages from lacerations of the cardiac orifice of the stomach due to vomiting. Am. J. Med. Sci. *178*: 506, 1929.

(17) Lynch, J. P.: Spontaneous perforation of the esophagus. N.E.J. Med. *241*: 395, 1949.

(18) Russell, J. Y. W.: Spontaneous perforation of the esophagus. Brit. J. Surg. *40*: 312, 1952–53.

(19) Dressler, W.: Percussion of the sternum. I. Aid to differentiation of pericardial effusion and cardiac dilatation. J.A.M.A. *173*: 761, 1960.

(20) Effler, D. B. and Proudfit, W. L.: Pericardial biopsy. Am. Rev. Tuberc. *75*: 469, 1957.

(21) Baird, J. and Prior, I.: Acute idiopathic pericarditis. Report of a case which progressed to chronic constrictive pericarditis requiring relief by pericardiectomy. New Zealand Med. J. *56*: 124, 1957.

(22) Tietze, A.: Ueber eine eigenartige Häufung von Fällen

mit Dystrophie der Rippenknorpel. Berliner Klin. Wchn-schr. *584*: 829, 1921.

(23) Wehrmacher, W. H.: Significance of Tietze's syndrome in differential diagnosis of chest pain. J.A.M.A. *157*: 505, 1955.

(24) Motulsky, A. G. and Rohn, R. J.: Tietze's syndrome, cause of chest pain and chest wall swelling. J.A.M.A. *152*: 504, 1953.

(25) Benson, E. H. and Zavala, D. C.: Importance of costo-chondral syndrome in evaluation of chest pain. Report of 62 cases. J.A.M.A. *156*: 1244, 1954.

(26) Prinzmetal, M. and Massumi, R. A.: The anterior chest wall syndrome—Chest pain resembling pain of cardiac origin. J.A.M.A. *159*: 177, 1955.

(27) Miller, A. J. and Texidor, T. A.: "Precordial catch," a neg-lected syndrome of precordial pain. J.A.M.A. *159*: 1364, 1955.

(28) Palmer, E. D.: Hiatus hernia in the adult. Clinical mani-festations. Am. J. Dig. Dis. *3*: 45, 1958.

(29) Benedict, E. B. and Sweet, R. H.: Benign stricture of the esophagus with special reference to esophagitis, hiatus hernia, esophageal ulcer, and duodenal ulcer. Gastroen-terology *11*: 618, 1948.

5

PULMONARY EMBOLISM, PULMONARY INFARCTION AND ACUTE COR PULMONALE

Clinical Syndrome

Physical Examination

Laboratory Findings

Importance of Leg Vein Thrombosis

Treatment-General Measures

Anticoagulant Therapy

Vein Ligation

5

PULMONARY EMBOLISM,

PULMONARY INFARCTION

AND ACUTE COR PULMONALE

Until fairly recently pulmonary embolism was considered to be a complication developing pre-eminently in post-operative or post-partum patients. Extensive post-mortem studies indicate, however, that well over half of cases of pulmonary emoblism in large metropolitan hospitals are observed on the medical wards and affect particularly patients with heart disease.[1,2,3] Before proceeding to a description of the symptomatology, the three distinct entities listed in the title of this chapter deserve definition. *Pulmonary infarction* indicates consolidation of an area of pulmonary tissue due to occlusion of the pulmonary artery branch which supplies it. This is generally the result of lodgement of an embolus in that artery ("pulmonary embolism") but in rare cases it may be due to primary thrombosis beginning *de novo* in that artery. Where it is embolic the fragment of clot may have been detached from thrombi in the leg veins or in the vena cava or its intrapelvic tributaries (94.4%), in very rare instances from a dilated or fibrillating right auricle, or from a mural thrombus in the right ventricle.[3] *Acute cor pulmonale* represents the cardiovascular response to an acute overloading of the right side of the heart. Pulmonary infarction may occur together with or in the absence of acute cor pulmonale. Acute cor pulmonale is generally, but not necessarily, the result of pulmonary embolism; but at times it may be induced by other causes such as acute pneumonia, acute pulmonary edema, bronchial asthma or massive collapse of the lungs. Let it be said at the outset that the diagnosis of these conditions is difficult and, of necessity, frequently tenuous. As viewed in retrospect by the pathologist, the clinical course of fatal pulmonary embolism is diverse. In one group death is sudden and unexpected and often misdiagnosed at the bedside as the result of coronary occlusion. In a second group a subacute pattern is exhibited with a protracted terminal illness lasting days or weeks and frequently misinterpreted as bronchopneumonia. And finally there is a "chronic" or "recurrent" group of patients who die quietly after a long illness with minimal respiratory symptoms.[4]

CLINICAL SYNDROME

The clinical picture produced by pulmonary embolism apparently depends upon the size of the dislodged thrombus, the size of the occluded artery, the existent degree of pulmonary congestion and upon the resultant degree of overburdening of the right ventricle. If the main pulmonary artery becomes occluded the patient dies rapidly, generally after an agony of five or ten minutes. The same sequence may occur with occlusion of the right or left pulmonary artery or of two or three of the subdivisions of each.[5] Pulmonary infarction is not induced by occlusion of the right or left pulmonary artery or of the first subdivisions of the lobar branches. Occlusion at this level, if not fatal, gives rise to the clinical picture of acute cor pulmonale. It is only when the smaller, peripheral branches are occluded that the symptoms and signs of pulmonary infarction develop. The patient complains of the sudden onset of severe pain in the chest which he may liken to "being struck by a steam-roller." The pain becomes pleuritic in type and may be associated with painful cough and frank hemoptysis, or the raising of bloody sputum. The obstetrician is prone to assume the development of pulmonary embolism when the post-partem chart shows a sharp rise in temperature, particularly if there is a simultaneous rise in pulse and respiration (Allen's sign). This triad of brisk fever, panting tachypnea and tachycardia deserve equally the attention of the internist and general practitioner. One will be loathe to make the diagnosis of pulmonary embolism unless there is a respectable degree of tachycardia. Among medical patients these symptoms may develop on a background of pre-existent congestive heart failure; here there may be merely an accentuation of symptoms already present. Occasionally pulmonary infarction is associated with profuse sweating, shock or pulmonary edema. Thus either shock or pulmonary edema, or the two in combination, may constitute the presenting evidence of pulmonary infarction. It is not clear to what extent certain of these conditions, particularly tachycardia, tachypnea, shock and pulmonary edema, are the consequences of pulmonary infarction *per se* or require the simultaneous operation of acute cor pulmonale.

In certain rapidly fatal cases of pulmonary embolism meticulous pathological examination shows only a small embolus in one of the finer radicles of the pulmonary artery. Yet the patient is just as dead as if he had had a straddle embolus in the main pulmonary artery. It has been assumed by some authorities that obstruction of one of these small arteries or even arterioles is capable of setting up spasm of the collateral pulmonary arteries intense enough to induce a severe grade of hypertension in the pulmonary circuit thus overwhelming the right ventricle. Such pulmonary hypertension is apparently part and parcel of the syndrome of acute cor pulmonale. This gives rise to the abrupt development or exaggeration of right-sided congestive heart failure. It may also produce a pain which is not at all pleuritic in type. It is described rather as a substernal or precordial angina-like or pressure pain. The patient, if he has previously suffered with angina pectoris, may insist upon the resemblance of this pain to his angina. The duration of the pain may even suggest acute myocardial infarction. The difficulty is compounded by the fact that myocardial infarction is not infrequently complicated by the development of pulmonary embolism and that, in rare instances, pulmonary embolism may even be complicated by the superimposed development of myocardial infarction. There is experimental and, as we shall see, electrocardiographic evidence that such pain occurring in acute cor pulmonale is in fact due to associated acute coronary insufficiency. Certain symptoms referable to the central nervous system may also be manifestations of acute cor pulmonale, e.g. dizziness, faintness, convulsions or syncope.[6] The latter may be related to abruptly developing hypertension in the pulmonary artery, perhaps by a mechanism akin to the so-called "tussive syncope" described on page 321.

PHYSICAL EXAMINATION

In pulmonary infarction physical examination may disclose findings suggesting pneumonia. The chest may be "splinted" at one lung base or the other and breath sounds suppressed in the same locality. A leathery friction rub may be heard in this area. The classical evidence of pulmonary consolidation—bronchial breathing and fine to medium crackling râles—may be heard with the stethoscope. There may also be signs of effusion into either pleural space; this effusion is apt to be bloody. Not infrequently the patient with pulmonary infarction exhibits slight to moderate or, in rare cases, even extreme jaundice.

[118]

As a consequence of acute cor pulmonale the neck veins may become acutely distended, or, if already distended, more so. The liver may become palpable and tender or, if already palpable, larger. The pulmonic second sound may become accentuated. Rarely a particularly accomplished clinician may be able to percuss an area of dullness in the second and third intercostal spaces just to the left of the sternum; this finding suggests dilatation of the pulmonary artery. Or a systolic or to-and-fro friction rub may be heard in the same locality or over a larger area of distribution. This may be attributable to contact of the dilated pulmonary artery with the inner surface of the chest wall or with other structures. In the uncomplicated case it is not due to pericarditis for a pericardial reaction is not demonstrable at autopsy.

The physical findings are extraordinarily variable. In some patients examination is quite negative or shows nothing not previously noted save some increase in the heart rate. Others may show all of the physical stigmata just enumerated. The findings take on increased significance when compared with the original examination. For example, the finding of an accentuated pulmonic second sound would be more impressive if it is known that the aortic second sound was previously louder than the pulmonic second sound. And dullness in the second and third interspace would mean more if this area were previously resonant. The timing of the clinical episode in relation to previous surgery may be of some help in the diagnosis. In healthy individuals recovering normally after surgery this complication generally occurs between the fourth and tenth days but in patients with pre-existent congestive heart failure, cancer, sepsis, leg vein disease, fractures of the legs, renal shutdown, electrolyte imbalance or wound dehiscence, the evidence of embolism may appear quite promptly after surgery.

LABORATORY FINDINGS

Laboratory examination may show a leucocytosis or an elevated icteric index or bilirubin level. Certain serum enzyme concentrations, such as the serum transaminase and lactic acid dehydrogenase, may be slightly to moderately elevated but do not attain the extremely high levels observed in some cases of acute myocardial infarction. Roentgen-ray examination of the chest and electrocardiograms are generally much more helpful than these laboratory examinations. A bedside portable X-ray examination is of little value. If at all feasible, the patient, if hospitalized, should be taken in his bed to the X-ray Department where a creditable chest film can be made. Because the area of consolidation is more frequently located in the lower than in the upper lobes and may be tucked behind the cardiac silhouette, this should include postero-anterior and lateral films, oblique films or a stereoroentgenogram. At times pencils of rays beamed to the lower lung regions in over-exposed films may bring out areas otherwise poorly visualized or not seen at all. If the condition of the patient does not justify his removal to the X-Ray Department, reliance may have to be placed upon a bedside film or a decision made without benefit of X-rays.

We are indebted to Fleischner [7] for a description of the entire roentgenologic spectrum of pulmonary embolism. He points out that the pulmonary infarct is roughly hemispherical with its longest diameter plastered against a pleural surface whether this is at the lung surface or at the interlobar, diaphragmatic or mediastinal pleura. Careful positioning may be necessary at fluoroscopy to localize the infarct. The pulmonary lesion may be a conical affair, wedge-shaped when seen in profile, rounded when seen end-on, but this appearance is very much the exception rather than the rule. It is more commonly cushion-shaped or hemispherical. Early in the course of the infarction it is generally poorly defined; later it may become more sharply delineated. (Fig. 8,C.) As a result of poor aeration of a lower lobe the diaphragm may occupy a position higher than normal. This may be indicated by a diminished distance from the horizontal interlobar fissure to the diaphragm. This finding may be unilateral or bilateral. Frequently even an experienced roentgenologist can do no more than venture the opinion that there is one or more than one poorly defined area of consolidation, congestion or infiltration compatible with pneumonia or pulmonary infarct. As the infarct heals it shrinks to form a flat, fibrotic streak just beneath the pleura, resembling an area of plate-like atelectasis. It differs from the latter in that it is usually shorter, it may end in a nodular extremity, it is disposed in a single plane and it may run in any direction.[8] The difficulty may be compounded by the fact that these scars may be associated with actual areas of atelectasis. The X-ray is much more helpful in purely surgical than in medical cases. It is said to reveal convincing evidence in about half of patients in the former category, in about a quarter of patients with heart disease.

Fleishner has emphasized that X-ray examination may show not only evidence of pulmonary infarction but of acute pulmonary hypertension ("acute cor pulmonale") as well. This consists of increased translucency of a pneumonic or lobar lung field and of dilatation of the hilar arteries into plump, tumor-like shadows. The former change is attributable to oligemia from spasm of the more muscular peripheral arteries, the latter to dilatation of the more elastic central arteries. Increased back-pressure may be reflected in dilatation of the superior vena cava and the azygos vein.

The electrocardiogram may show any of a number of features, isolated or in combination, transiently or persistently. An S wave may develop in Lead I (Fig. 8,B) or a Q wave in Lead III, neither previously present or, if present previously, they be-

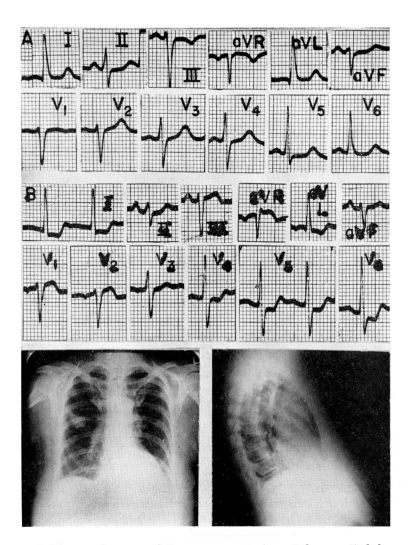

Fig. 8. *Electrocardiogram and Roentgenogram in Acute Pulmonary Embolism.* (A) Normal pre-operative electrocardiogram in 67-year-old woman with thrombophlebitis whose right saphenous vein was ligated on November 10, 1955. Heparin started three days later when she developed left calf tenderness. Episode of chest pain and syncope while at stool November 19 while heparin being tapered. Friction rub and neck vein distension. Bilateral common femoral vein ligation that evening; clot found in left common femoral vein, none on right. X-rays November 23 showed increased markings at right lung base. (B) EKG recorded November 27 showing heart rate 110, prominent S_1 and depressed RS-T segments in Leads I, II, aVL and V_4 through V_6. (Below) X-rays next day showing emergence of sharply demarcated cone-shaped infiltration in right mid-lung field previously poorly defined. Caval ligation three days later with uneventful recovery and total clearing of lungs.

[122]

come more prominent. To this extent acute cor pulmonale may resemble acute diaphragmatic myocardial infarction. It has been claimed that under these circumstances a significant Q wave does not develop in Lead aVF. This is true in most cases but does not enable one to make the differentiation with complete assurance. The so-called "transitional zone" may migrate to the left, even beyond precordial position V$_6$. Small shifts of, say, one or two positions, are unimpressive evidence for this diagnosis since slight changes in the electrical position of the heart can develop for many other reasons than acute cor pulmonale. This change should be accorded very little weight in the diagnosis of acute cor pulmonale unless the heart rate is rapid at the same time. The T waves may become smartly inverted over the right precordium and occasionally the RS-T segments slightly elevated in the same leads. Acute antero-septal infarction may thus be simulated. The RS-T segments may become sharply depressed over the left precordium (Fig. 8,B) or over the entire precordium and sometimes in certain extremely leads as well. The appearance has been likened to a "staircase ascent," [9] resembles the RS-T shift seen in a "positive" Master test, and presumably indicates subendocardial ischemia. Transient complete or, more commonly, incomplete, right bundle branch block may also be detected. It may require frequent and repetitive tracings to pick up these changes. The P waves may become prominent. The electrocardiogram may, in rare cases, give the first clue to the development of acute cor pulmonale. It must be remembered, on the other hand, that electrocardiographic changes are recorded in only a minority of patients with this syndrome.

IMPORTANCE OF LEG VEIN THROMBOSIS

As helpful in the diagnosis as these physical and laboratory findings may be, they mean little alongside the detection of a seeding source for these emboli. In medical patients in general, and cardiac patients in particular, these emboli arise in the leg veins in the overwhelming majority of cases.[2,10,11] A diligent and deliberate search must therefore be made in these patients for evidence of thrombophlebitis. Each and all of the following findings suggest the presence of thrombophlebitis in the leg and are strong evidence, in association with a suspect history, for pulmonary embolism: the detection of tenderness or deep induration in either calf, of tenderness over the femoral vessels or over the great saphenous vein, of pain induced in the leg by inflation of a blood pressure cuff about the calf, of involuntary resistance to forced dorsiflexion of the patient's foot (Homans' sign), or of an increasing circumference of the calf or thigh, as determined by careful daily and routinely recorded measurements made with a tape measure at a certain definite distance from the patella. This measurement will, of course, be more significant in patients without congestive heart failure and those who have not worn elastic stockings or bandages. On the other hand, the absence of demonstrable objective evidence of thrombophlebitis does not necessarily rule out either thrombophlebitis or pulmonary embolism. One must be willing at times to assume the existence of thrombophlebitis when there is clear-cut evidence of pulmonary embolism. By the same token, one must be willing to assume the existence or imminence of pulmonary embolism when there is convincing evidence of thrombophlebitis. Particularly in this category of patients with congestive heart failure or recent myocardial infarction who are doing poorly, one must furthermore be willing to accept the existence of both embolism and thrombophlebitis when there is no proof of either. And, finally, one must also assume that the process of thrombophlebitis is bilateral even though the signs of this condition are demonstrable in only one leg or, for that matter, in neither leg.

TREATMENT—GENERAL MEASURES

Treatment has two purposes—the relief of the immediate symptoms and, much more important, the prevention of further, and possibly fatal embolism. The first of these purposes may be fulfilled by the use of morphine, oxygen and atropine in full therapeutic dosage. In the case of atropine this is 1 to 2 mgms; therapeutic doses of papaverine have been recommended but its alleged value as an antagonist to spasm in the collateral pulmonary vasculature remains questionable. Phlebotomy should not wittingly be done in this emergency for it may accentuate an existent coronary insufficiency which, as we have seen, may be an integral feature of acute cor pulmonale. Removal of a thrombus from the common pulmonary artery (Trendelenburg operation) is spectacular but generally futile. We have recently seen the first successful American case.[12]

ANTICOAGULANT THERAPY

The two principal forms of preventive treatment are anticoagulant therapy and ligation of effluent veins. A prolonged controversy continues between the medical proponents of the former and the surgical champions of the latter. When the diagnosis is merely tentative and is unsupported by confirmatory laboratory or physical findings the inclination will be to anticoagulant therapy. Anticoagulants have the theoretical advantages of diminishing rather than adding to the extent of venous block in the leg veins, and of reducing the tendency to propagation of thrombi in leg veins, right heart and pulmonary arteries.[13] In this situation the possibility of surgery always lurks in the background. Furthermore the prolonged clotting time induced by heparin can be more rapidly and certainly abbreviated by the use of protamine than can the hypoprothrombinemia induced by dicumarol be eliminated by Vitamin K$_1$ oxide. Therefore preference will be given to heparin. This treatment should be continued for from 7 to 10 days and until the patient has become ambulatory. If one chooses to embark upon long-term therapy, dicumarol will be preferred.

As in the case of acute myocardial infarction, fibrinolysin therapy may eventually deserve a place in any consideration of the management of these vascular pulmonary emergencies. At present such a discussion would be premature.

VEIN LIGATION

Where the diagnosis of pulmonary embolism is clear-cut, and this is patently related to thrombophlebitis in the leg veins, particularly if pulmonary emboli persist during optimal anticoagulant therapy, the femoral veins should be ligated on both sides. This procedure is attended with the risk of hemorrhage and hematoma formation, particularly if anticoagulant therapy is resumed immediately after surgery. In rare cases a lymph fistula may develop and become secondarily infected. Emboli may continue to seed from the legs when only the superficial femoral veins are tied. Therefore the common rather than the superficial femoral veins should be ligated. This entails the risk that persistent edema of the legs may eventually develop. This possibility should be explained to the patient or to her family, especially if she is a young woman. In this situation the risk attendant on not operating may much more than overbalance this potential hazard. Ligation of the common femoral vein above the point of entrance of the deep femoral vein but below the points of entrance of all, or most, lateral and medial femoral circumflex veins has the merit of not trapping such large amounts of blood.[14] The use of this technique has minimized postoperative swelling.[15]

If the patient has been receiving coumarin or phenanedione anticoagulants before operation, these should be discontinued. If the patient has been receiving heparin, this should be interrupted. At the time of ligation the surgeon should note carefully whether thrombi are seen in the veins or whether "back bleeding" is diminished. This serves as a partial check on the diagnosis, may help explain subsequent edema and may influence the decision regarding further surgery. Thus persistence of pulmonary symptoms after the ligation of demonstrably thrombosed veins may be warrant for ligation of the inferior vena cava. If no thrombi are observed at the time of the original ligation, but the patient improves only later to re-develop symptoms, caval ligation may be performed but this would be of less certain value.

Where the source of embolism is uncertain, it is wise to initiate or resume anticoagulants after surgery despite the risk of hematoma formation. This may diminish thrombosis below the ligature, prevent thrombosis proximal to the ligature and "cover" other possible sources of embolism. Heparin can be started immediately after surgery.

In cases where an absolute or relative contraindication exists to the use of anticoagulants, continued embolism to the lungs or elsewhere may force one's hand to this form of treatment. As an alternative or as an adjunct to anticoagulants elastic stockings or bandages [16,17] may be snugly applied to the legs from feet to knees. By increasing the flow in the deep veins, these prevent local stagnation of blood and intravascular thrombosis. The general tendency is to apply these stockings too tightly. Since this may injure the skin at the upper edge of the stocking it may well do more harm than good. For most individuals a large size stocking is therefore preferable. For those with very large legs an "extra large" size is available. Ace binders three or four inches wide have the advantage of being adaptable to the size and contour of any leg but they tend to unravel and require frequent and generally neglected re-application. Stockings or binders should not be used in patients with evidence of significant arterial insufficiency.

REFERENCES

(1) Carlotti, J., Hardy, I. B., Jr., Linton, H. R. and White, P. D.: Pulmonary embolism in medical patients. J.A.M.A. *134*: 1447, 1947.

(2) Byrne, J. J. and O'Neill, E. E.: Fatal pulmonary emboli: a study of 130 autopsy-proven fatal emboli. Am. J. Surg. *83*: 47, 1952.

(3) Zeitlhofer, J. and Reiffenstuhl, G.: Untersuchungen über fulminante, tödliche, Lungenembolien am Obduktionsma-terial der Jahre 1941 bis 1951. Wien. Klin. Wchnschr. *64*: 446, 1952.

(4) Towbin, A.: Pulmonary embolism. Incidence and signifi-cance. J.A.M.A. *156*: 209, 1954.

(5) Crane, C.: Personal communication.

(6) Sagall, E. L., Bornstein, J. and Wolff, L.: Clinical syn-drome in patients with pulmonary embolism. Arch. Int. Med. *76*: 234, 1945.

(7) Fleischner, F. G.: Pulmonary embolism. The Louis Gross Memorial Address. Canad. Med. Ass'n. J. *78*: 653, 1958.

(8) Fleischner, F., Hampton, A. O. and Castleman, B.: Lin-ear shadows in the lung (Interlobar pleuritis, atelectasis and healed infarction). Am. J. Roentgen. *46*: 610, 1941.

(9) McGinn, S. and White, P. D.: Acute cor pulmonale re-sulting from pulmonary embolism. Its clinical recognition. J.A.M.A. *104*: 1473, 1935.

(10) Cohn, R. and Walsh, J.: The incidence and anatomical

site of origin of pulmonary emboli. Stanford Med. Bull. 4: 97, 1946.

(11) Short, D. S.: A survey of pulmonary embolism in a general hospital. Brit. Med. J. 1: 790, 1952.

(12) Steenberg, R. W., Warren, R., Wilson, R. E. and Rudolf, L. E.: Pulmonary embolectomy: a new look at an old operation. S.G.O. 107: 214, 1958.

(13) Crane, C.: Deep venous thrombosis and pulmonary embolism. Experience with 391 patients treated with heparin and 126 patients treated by venous division, with a review of the literature. N.E.J. Med. 257: 147, 1957.

(14) Edwards, E. A. and Robuck, J. D.: Applied anatomy of the femoral vein and its tributaries. S.G.O. 85: 547, 1947.

(15) Edwards, E. A.: Personal communication.

(16) Wilkins, R. W., Mixter, G., Jr., Stanton, J. R. and Litter, J.: Elastic stockings in prevention of pulmonary embolism: a preliminary report. N.E.J. Med. 246: 360, 1952.

(17) Wilkins, R. W. and Stanton, J. R.: Elastic stockings in prevention of pulmonary embolism: A progress report. N.E.J. Med. 248: 1087, 1953.

CHAPTER

6

"REFRACTORY" CONGESTIVE HEART FAILURE

Review of Diagnosis

Review of Treatment

Use of Mechanical Measures

Malabsorption of Digitalis

Electrolyte Imbalance

Tandem Diuretic Therapy

Steroid Therapy

Optimism in Therapy

CHAPTER

6

"REFRACTORY" CONGESTIVE

HEART FAILURE

To discuss this subject involves a deliberate departure
from the practice, thus far followed, of considering only
topics commonly accepted as acute cardiac emergencies.
Abrupt failure of the left ventricle with flooding of the lungs
is a dramatic clinical event. Though it is argued whether such
conditions as "pure" left ventricular failure or "pure" right ventricular failure actually exist, right-sided failure is commonly
regarded as manifesting hepatic enlargement, congestion of
the neck veins, dependent edema, anasarca and elevation of
the venous pressure. Characteristically, this condition develops
more insidiously than left ventricular failure and the patient
in whom right heart failure is a predominant or sôle feature
does not appear to be as obviously imperilled or to present the
urgent need for immediate action that is demanded in acute
pulmonary edema. In general, this syndrome is well treated;
its management with digitalis, depletion measures and rest is too
well-recognized to deserve repetition here. There are certain
times, however, when the patient, at the outset or later, is,
or becomes, resistant to measures which are ordinarily effective.
This is currently referred to as "refractoriness" to therapy. Such
refractoriness could be defined in several ways, for example,

in terms of difficulty in slowing the heart, in lowering the venous pressure or in eliminating edema. It is in the latter sense that this term will be used through this chapter. While not an emergency of the spectacular urgency of many of the conditions already enumerated, these individuals nonetheless may, over a longer period of time, present some of the less dramatic considerations outlined in the introductory chapter. This discussion will be limited to a consideration of certain aspects of this problem which seem commonly to be neglected. There is a general tendency to attribute this failure to respond to an unrecognized complex or esoteric disturbance such as electrolyte imbalance. Actually such an explanation is rarely an early or first consideration. The difficulty may be rather an error in the original diagnosis or some simple flaw in management.

REVIEW OF DIAGNOSIS

The first step is a thoroughgoing review of the diagnosis. Two diagnoses must be made: first that of the underlying heart disease; second, that of the precipitating factor which has thrust the previously well-compensated individual into congestive heart failure. For each of these categories, fundamental cause and triggering mechanism, one must be particularly alert to the possibility of having missed a curable or reversible condition. The review must not be reluctant, perfunctory or casual, but a sincere re-appraisal of all facts or clues available in the original or, if necessary, in a revised clinical history, in the physical examination or in the data supplied by various laboratory examinations or special procedures. The physician must be ready and willing to re-question patient, family and previous medical attendants, any one of whom may be able to supply information which is decisive to a correct diagnosis.

To spell out this habit of thinking in extensive detail is beyond the scope of this book. No simple formula can be advanced. Among precipitating factors one must consider pulmonary embolism, sodium indiscretion, arrhythmias, anemia, myocardial infarction, occult active rheumatic carditis, subacute bacterial endocarditis and extracardiac infections such as acute bronchitis or viral pneumonitis. Among primary cardiac diagnoses, particular thought should be directed to thyrotoxicosis, constrictive pericarditis, "pure" and operable mitral stenosis and such congenital cardiac defects as patent ductus arteriosus, coarctation of the aorta and atrial septal defect.

REVIEW OF TREATMENT

One must also review previous and current therapy. The order book and cardex should be thoroughly scrutinized. The physican will often be embarrassed to discover that some medication had not been ordered or discontinued as he had intended it to be. Even when all orders have been properly written, it is important at this time of urgency to clear the decks and rid the order sheet of all superfluous medication. This applies particularly to barbiturates, vitamins, "favorite drugs" and proprietary preparations of unproved or dubious value. Furthermore if a drug has been given for a specific purpose and it has not accomplished that purpose in the dosage prescribed, either the dose should be increased or, if this is not advisable or safe, the drug omitted altogether. This means that quinidine might well be omitted if given as a prophylaxis against arrhythmias if these arrhythmias are not clearly prevented by its use. Queer mental states developing at this time, often glibly referred to as "cardiac psychoses," may indeed be due to the grave cardiac disease [1] and to resultant cerebral anoxia or edema, or to digitalis intoxication [2,3,4] or to ammonium intoxication,[5,6] but a first consideration will be to discontinue all barbiturates as a more likely cause of these symptoms.

All other things being equal, it is desirable to have these difficult patients in the hospital. Very often the mere change from the home to the hospital environment, with little if any other change in management, may coincide with the beginning improvement of the patient. Here optimal rest and rigid salt restriction, previously enjoined and assumed but not really practiced, are actually put into effect. Desirable as this is, it is, unfortunately, not always feasible. Congestive heart failure is generally a long-term business, subject to repeated exacerbation. Often the patient will have exhausted his hospitalization insurance coverage or, as a consequence of repeated hospitalizations, have been converted from a solvent to a bankrupt individual. In such cases one may have to manage as well as one can with home care.

USE OF MECHANICAL MEASURES

Even when the underlying diagnosis has been correctly made, the tide may still be turned by the timely use of one or more simple mechanical measures. Thus the detection and removal of a previously unsuspected pleural effusion or the correction of an appreciable hypervolemia by a phlebotomy may yet mark the turning point in the downhill course of congestive failure. This precedure may deserve a trial even if the blood pressure or hematocrit level is not elevated. The removal of a hardly appreciated accumulation of ascitic fluid may relieve the increased intraabdominal pressure coming to bear upon the kidneys and now make them respond with a brisk diuresis to doses of mercurial diuretics which have hitherto been ineffective. Massive edema of the legs may be relieved by the insertion of Southey's tubes under the subcutaneous tissue on the median and lateral aspects of the dorsum of each foot. These tubes are inserted under aseptic precautions and connected through small-bore rubber tubes (ureteral catheters, for example) to a bottle under the bed, through a Y tube. The fluid is allowed to siphon off over the course of 6 to 10 hours, while the patient is in bed. Here again a subsequent diuretic may prove effective where it had been ineffective before the mechanical drainage.

There is another mechanical aspect of the treatment of congestive heart failure. This has been emphasized by S. A. Levine [7,8] and concerns the benefits to be derived from having the patient sitting up in a comfortable chair rather than lying flat in bed. Among the advantages of the sitting, over the recumbent posture, are an increased vital capacity of the lungs, a decrease in the venous return to the heart, a decrease in cardiac work, a redistribution of fluid from chest to legs by gravity resulting in a decrease in the degree of pulmonary edema and in the tendency to complicating pneumonia, easier bladder function, prevention of asthenia, brightening and shortening of convalescence and improvement in the patient's comfort and morale. The recumbent posture, on the other hand, produces hemodilution, increases the effective blood volume and the work of the heart and encourages urinary retention and secondary urinary tract infections.[7] It leads to the development of bedsores and induces constipation and straining at stool and is therefore often responsible for bedpan deaths. Elderly patients in congestive heart failure are particularly prone to these risks. In short, the upright position provides a greater degree of physiological rest for the ailing heart. Having the patient propped up in his bed is better than having him lie down but, by and large, it is not so satisfactory as having him up in a chair. With the patient in bed it is difficult to have him seated bolt upright. His legs are not down. And he tends to slump down from his original position.

These considerations are pertinent when the patient is first seen early in the course of his acute congestive heart failure. Many patients treated by orthodox rest in bed will nonetheless have done well; these present no problem. But in the patient who has been treated over a long period of time in the tradi-

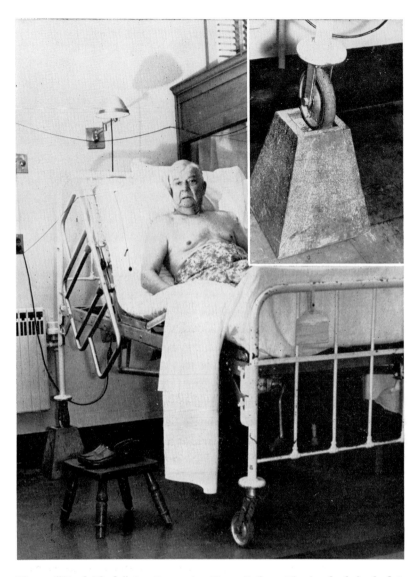

Fig. 9. *"Head Blocks" for Congestive Heart Failure.* The head of the bed is elevated on pyramidal blocks 6 to 10 inches high (here 9 inches), slanting the entire bed from head to foot. Additional elevation may be attained by cranking up the head of the bed and using several pillows. Sliding down is avoided by cranking up foot of bed, flexing knees and jackknifing trunk and by use of footboard. Inset shows detail of one type of bed block.

[138]

tional fashion, who has done poorly, who is literally drowning in his own pulmonary secretions and seems to be in extremis, these considerations are even more pertinent. The patient's condition is then truly an acute medical emergency. Getting him forthrightly out of bed into a chair may now over a short period of time produce a dramatic improvement in his condition.

There is an entirely understandable reluctance on the part of physicians to initiate this, by current standards, unorthodox form of therapy. They fear the censure of other physicians and of relatives in the event of a fatality, a fatality which might well have been inevitable if the patient were kept in bed. In effect, if the patient dies flat, all is forgiven; if he dies sitting up in a chair, the physician is blamed for his demise. Keeping the desperately ill decompensated patient in bed may therefore preserve the unsullied reputation of his attending physician; but it doesn't help the patient. Except for patients in obvious shock the arm-chair treatment is strongly recommended. In getting the patient out of bed it is neither necessary nor advisable that he be lifted bodily. There is probably more work involved on the part of the patient in clumsily holding onto the attendant than in getting out on his own power while being assisted. The patient is therefore first placed in a sitting position at the edge of the bed, a stool is placed at his feet and he is literally guided onto the stool and floor, then into the chair. The chair should be comfortably padded, its back fairly straight, and it should be supplied with a support for head and arms. (Fig. 10). The legs should hang straight down. The patient should be encouraged to remain up in the chair for as long as he feels comfortable in it. As soon as he becomes tired he should be returned to bed in a reverse manner. If this treatment is started early the patient often notes a return of his muscle tone within a day or two. *It must be made clear to the attendants and physicians that he is not being ambulated.* He is merely allowed up in the chair

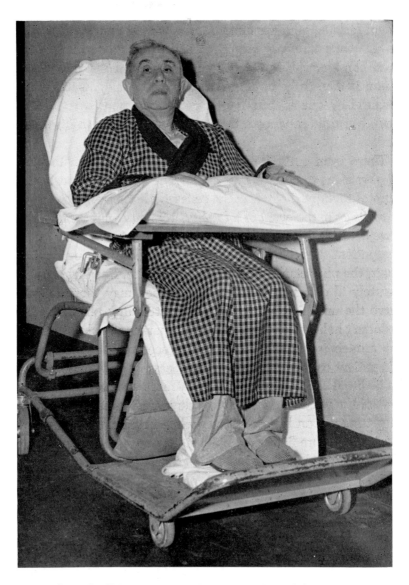

Fig. 10. *"Armchair"* for treatment of congestive heart failure or acute myocardial infarction. The patient is seated comfortably in a well-padded chair
with head and arms supported. This position provides maximal physiological
rest for the ailing heart.

and must not walk about the ward to visit other patients or to use the lavatory.

MALABSORPTION OF DIGITALIS

There are differences in the degree to which different digitalis glycosides are taken up from the gastrointestinal tract. Thus digitoxin is said to be completely, digoxin fairly completely, absorbed. We often forget that absorption is a function of other variables than the particular glycoside used. Among other factors, the absorption of digitalis from the intestinal tract is dependent upon the functional integrity of the bowel mucosa. When the bowel mucosa is edematous a smaller proportion of the offered medication is accepted. Digitoxin would not then be "100% absorbed;" instead smaller proportions, even none whatever, will be removed from the gastrointestinal tract. There is nothing new about this. Before the advent of the newer injectable digitalis glycosides it was customary to instill an infusion of digitalis as a retention enema in patients whose hearts failed to slow on oral digitalis. With this technique either absorption is better or the drug has a more prolonged contact with mucosa. At any rate this departure from the usual therapy frequently produced a gratifying response when much larger oral doses had been ineffective. The same purpose can now be accomplished by shifting from an oral to an intravenous or intramuscular preparation. I have seen this accomplished in patients with atrial fibrillation and rapid ventricular rate by simply shifting from oral to intramuscular digitoxin in unchanged dosage. Patients receiving 0.2 mgm. daily for weeks or months often slowed within three days when they were given identical amounts of digitoxin intramuscularly. Where more rapid effect is necessary digoxin may be given intravenously.

ELECTROLYTE IMBALANCE

A number of derangements in electrolyte balance and water metabolism can result in refractoriness to the measures usually employed in the treatment of heart failure. These may occur spontaneously as a result of the underlying disease state or as a result of therapy. Before proceeding to a review of these derangements a few general statements regarding electrolyte balance are in order. The concentration of cations (sodium, potassium, calcium, magnesium) must equal the concentration of anions (bicarbonate, chloride, phosphate, sulfate, organic acids, proteinate) in the extracellular fluid. These values were formerly expressed in milligrams per cent. But it is much simpler and more meaningful to express the values in milliequivalents per liter. Allowing for differences in valence, the sum total of cation in milliequivalents must equal the sum total of anion in milliequivalents. As a practical matter it is ordinarily not necessary to determine the concentration of all ions. The determination of sodium, potassium, chloride and bicarbonate levels is usually enough. The normal serum sodium concentration is 142 mEq/l (milliequivalents per liter) with a range of 138 to 144. The normal serum bicarbonate is 27 (range 22–30) mM/l (millimols per liter) and the normal chloride 103 (range 99–111) mEq/l. Where a serum sodium level cannot be determined directly one may calculate the probable sodium value by adding 12 to the measured total of bicarbonate and chloride. It is to be emphasized that these figures refer to the *concentrations* of these ions and do not necessarily reflect changes in the total extracellular amounts of these ions. These figures thus give no indication of contraction or expansion of the total extracellular fluid volume. For a further exposition of this aspect of the subject the reader is referred to the excellent presentation of Davenport.[9]

Hypochloremic alkalosis   As a consequence of repeated mercurial diureses or of vomiting, large amounts of chloride ion may be lost in the urine or vomitus. This may result in a significant fall in the serum chloride level. This fall is accompanied by a concomitant rise in the serum bicarbonate level so that the total of chloride and bicarbonate remains unchanged. There is no change, or at most only a slight and unimportant fall in the serum sodium level. Many patients who show such a selective fall in chloride level now fail to respond to mercurial diuretics with a respectable diuresis.[10] Such a failure of response should not be met with a stubborn repetition of the mercurial. If it is found that the chloride level has fallen to, say, 94 mEq/l, a deliberate restoration of the chloride level to 100 or more mEq/l may now be followed by the same brisk diuresis previously exhibited. This non-responsiveness is probably a factor of acidity (pH) rather than of the chloride level per se. The threshold value for chloride in respect to the diuretic response apparently may vary somewhat, a level of 96 or 97 being quite adequate in some individuals; in others "pushing" the chloride to well over 100 may be necessary. This may be accomplished by giving (in solution, as enteric coated tablets or in gelatin capsules), ammonium chloride by mouth in doses of 1 to 2 grams three or four times daily. This syndrome of hypochloremic alkalosis may develop occasionally in patients receiving ammonium chloride in dosage inadequate to replace the large chloride losses accounted for by the large chloride content of the previously diuresed fluid, or in those who have been receiving but not absorbing chloride in routine continuous rations because of gastrointestinal intolerance or because the enteric coating is not broken down. It has recently been suggested that patients who have difficulty in handling the ammonium ion, may be treated effectively with lysine monohydrochloride. If the patient cannot tolerate large amounts of ammonium chloride by mouth, the chloride level may be restored by having the patient drink 20 cc. of U.S.P.

dilute hydrochloric acid diluted to a volume of 600 to 1000 cc. through a glass drinking tube. This can be made tolerably palatable by flavoring with syrup of wild cherry. As an alternative ammonium chloride may be given by vein. A 1% solution of ammonium chloride made up in a 5% solution of dextrose in water, given at a rate not exceeding 100 cc. per hour, is safe and may be effective. Ten to 15 grams may thus be given over the course of 24 hours.[10] But such heroic therapy will be only rarely necessary.

Hyperchloremic acidosis ("Ammonium chloride intoxication") Ammonium chloride should be given cautiously to patients with liver disease. The conversion of ammonium ion into urea depends upon the integrity of the liver cell. If ammonium chloride is given in too large a dose or too rapidly or over too long a period of time, this function of the liver may be overwhelmed, producing ammonia intoxication.[5,6,11] This is most apt to develop in patients with cardiac cirrhosis or congestive hepatomegaly but it may also occur in renal or pulmonary disease.

This condition is manifested by certain disturbances in the central nervous system, including weakness, lethargy, obtundation, semi-stupor, coma, delirium, clonic muscular jerkings and a specific tremor designated as the "hepatic flap."[12] This consists of a series of movements occurring when the patient stretches out his arms and hands and spreads his fingers apart. It includes lateral deviations of the fingers, flexion and extension of the fingers at the metacarpo-phalangeal joints and flexion-extension of the wrist, occurring at intervals varying from a fraction of a second to several seconds. A rough clinical guide to the severity of this disturbance may be furnished by the patient's handwriting. In ammonium chloride intoxication the respirations may be deep and sighing ("Kussmaul") in type and rapid. The carbon dioxide combining power (and carbon dioxide content) of the serum is low, the serum pH low, while

large losses of sodium from the body consequent upon sweating, vomiting or diarrhoea or from "salt-losing" nephritis. Considerable lowering of the serum sodium level may also develop during the phase of re-accumulation of fluid in the body spaces following the mechanical removal of large volumes of sodium-containing fluids (thoracentesis, abdominal paracentesis, Southey tube drainage, nasogastric suction, etc.), especially when these are replaced with water alone. Obviously each of these factors may operate alone or in various combinations. This syndrome may also be a dilution effect resulting from excessive retention of water ("water intoxication"). Post-operative cardiac patients and patients in renal failure and anuria are particularly disposed to this development especially if fluid is "forced."

Treatment depends upon the severity of the deficit and the condition of the patient. In some cases a relaxation in the stringency of salt restriction or perhaps the ingestion of bouillion (one cube contains $3\frac{1}{2}$ grams of salt) by mouth may be adequate.[13] Rarely it will be necessary to infuse hypertonic (3 to 5%) solution of sodium chloride by vein. If this is to be used at all, extreme caution must be exercised and the possibility of precipitating left ventricular failure anticipated. Generally one should plan to give the salt piecemeal over the course of three days or so rather than in a single day. The deficit is calculated by subtracting the determined serum sodium level in mEq/l from the normal of 142 mEq/l and multiplying by the total body water in kilograms (or 0.6 of the body weight in kilograms). This calculation is based upon total body water since it is the osmolality we are trying to raise. Thus if the serum sodium concentration is 122 mEq/l and the patient weighs 60 kilograms the deficit would be:

$$(142 - 122) \times (0.6 \times 60) = 20 \times 36 = 720 \text{ mEq}$$

Since one gram of sodium chloride equals 17 mEq of sodium chloride, the patient's deficit would be 42 grams. Giving 300 cc.

of 5% sodium chloride solution by slow intravenous infusion for two or three days would replace the deficit. Where clinical and chemical improvement does occur it generally develops fairly rapidly and on the initial infusion. Giving sodium to a potassium depleted patient may precipitate arrhythmias; therefore one should be certain that the patient is not also depleted of potassium before proceeding to replace only sodium. In those cases of low sodium syndrome which are associated with acidosis or with hyperchloremia one should give instead concentrated sodium bicarbonate or lactate by vein. Where the low sodium syndrome is the result of dilution, treatment is not the infusion of sodium chloride, but rigid restriction of the water intake. This injunction is particularly applicable in patients who show a transient fall in serum sodium and rise in potassium a few days postoperatively at a time when their total body sodium is actually normal.

TANDEM DIURETIC THERAPY. STEROID THERAPY

It is probable that the diuretic agents are effective in interfering with certain enzyme systems in the kidney. The idea has gained currency that some patients lose their responsiveness to a previously effective diuretic because the renal cell enzyme is no longer affected by this diuretic. On the theory that such altered responsiveness can be overwhelmed by concentrating not upon one, but, tandem fashion, upon a number of enzyme systems, the practice is becoming common, in such cases, to employ in sequence a number of different diuretic agents, each effective through a different mechanism. In one such regimen [14] one gives Diamox 250 mgms. b.i.d. for one day, Diuril 500 mgms. or Hydrodiuril 50 mgms. b.i.d. or t.i.d. for the next two days, then, perhaps, Neohydrin one tablet once or twice on the fourth day. The cycle is then repeated over the next four days and so on. Tandem therapy of this type is recommended as worthy of trial in difficult cases.

The so-called "merc-sandwich" is frequently very effective when other measures have failed. One gives 1 cc. of mercurial diuretic intramuscularly at 9 A.M. This is followed at 11 A.M. either by a slow infusion of 250 to 500 mgms. of aminophylline by vein or by the rectal installation of an aminophylline suppository. Then at 1 or 2 P.M. one injects another cc. of mercurial intramuscularly. It has recently been found that the continuous preparatory use of a spiro-lactone (aldosterone-inhibitor) enhances the effectiveness of a mercurial diuretic.[14] For this purpose one gives Aldactone 200 mgms. t.i.d. by mouth for four consecutive days. On the morning of the fourth day, while this preparation is still being given, one injects 2 cc. of mercurial diuretic i.m.

In desperate cases if the entire gamut of therapy outlined above has been exhausted and ineffective, steroid therapy may be tried. Certain compounds such as prednisolone (delta-1-hydrocortisone) and methyl prednisolone (6 methyl-delta-1-hydrocortisone) are now available which have relatively little sodium retaining activity. These corticosteroids potentiate the action of mercurial and carbonic anhydrase inhibiting diuretic agents. They appear to increase the glomerular filtration rate, to inhibit the adrenal production or action of aldosterone on tubular reabsorption of sodium and to oppose the action of posterior pituitary antidiuretic hormone. The recommended daily dose of prednisolone is 24 to 36 mgms., of methyl-prednisolone 16 to 24 mgms.[15] This should be divided into four doses, given one with each meal and one with a bedtime snack. Once an effect is attained, the decision must be made whether the medication is then to be stopped or to be continued in minimal effective maintenance dosage. The dose is tapered by 2 mgms. or so at 7 day intervals to a zero or maintenance level. The patient is observed most carefully during this period. The usual precautions for steroid therapy, particularly those pertaining to ulcer disease, tuberculosis, diabetes, psychoses and inter-current infection, must be rigidly observed. The possibility must be borne in mind of altered insulin requirement, of need for a high protein diet, for potassium supplementation or an anabolic agent.

OPTIMISM IN THERAPY

The patient with "refractory" failure, after attention has been paid to these various possibilities and appropriate corrections made, may continue to do badly. At this juncture the thought may occur to the physician that the underlying disease has simply progressed to the point where literally nothing more can be done. The patient, in short, has reached the end of his road! Such a hopeless point of view may be quite justified with regard to certain patients with cancer. And it must be conceded that there must be some heart patients in whom this may be true. But such an attitude should be strongly condemned when dealing with patients with "refractory" congestive failure. We can be so wrong when we think we are so right. The subsequent course of events so often shows the fallacy of the pessimistic diagnosis, and in fatal cases the findings at post-mortem so often disclose a remediable lesion, that one must always take the more aggressive and optimistic point of view and seek out the possibility that has not yet been considered.

REFERENCES

(1) Riesman, D.: Acute psychoses arising during the course of heart disease. Am. J. Med. Sci. *161*: 157, 1921.
(2) King, J. T.: Digitalis delirium. Ann. Int. Med. 33: 1360, 1950.

(3) Weiss, S.: Effects of digitalis bodies on the nervous system. M. Clin. No. Am. *15*: 963, 1932.

(4) Smith, H. L.: Cerebral manifestations of digitalis intoxication. Proc. Staff Meet. Mayo Clin. *13*: 574, 1938.

(5) Bessman, A. N. and Evans, J. M.: Blood ammonia in congestive heart failure. Am. Heart J. *50*: 715, 1955.

(6) Evans, J. M., Zimmerman, H. J., Wilmer, J. G., Thomas, L. J. and Ethridge, C. B.: Altered liver function of congestive heart failure. Am. J. Med. *13*: 704, 1952.

(7) Levine, S. A.: Some harmful effects of recumbency in the treatment of heart disease. J.A.M.A. *126*: 80, 1944.

(8) Levine, S. A. and Lown, B.: "Armchair" treatment of acute coronary thrombosis. J.A.M.A. *148*: 1365, 1952.

(9) Davenport, H. N.: The ABC of Acid-Base Chemistry. 4th Edition. University of Chicago Press, 1958.

(10) Schwartz, W. B. and Relman, A. S.: Electrolyte disturbances in congestive heart failure. Clinical significance and management. J.A.M.A. *154*: 1237, 1954.

(11) Robin, E. D.: Some hazards of ammonium chloride administration. (Unpublished data)

(12) Adams, R. D. and Foley, J. M.: The neurologic disorder associated with liver diseases. Arch. Nerv. and Ment. Dis. *32*: 198, 1953.

(13) Merrill, J. P.: The low salt syndrome. Modern Concepts Cardiovascular Disease, *24*: 283, 1955.

(14) Merrill, J. P.: Personal communication.

(15) Radó, J. P., Blumenfeld, G. and Hammer, S.: The effect of prednisone and 6-methyl-prednisolone on mercurial diuresis in patients with refractory cardiac edema. Am. J. Med. Sci. *238*: 542, 1959.

CHAPTER

7

OTHER ELECTROLYTE

DISTURBANCES AS

CARDIOVASCULAR

EMERGENCIES

Potassium   Intoxication

Potassium   Depletion

CHAPTER

7

OTHER ELECTROLYTE

DISTURBANCES AS

CARDIOVASCULAR

EMERGENCIES

In the preceding chapter we have considered a number of electrolyte derangements which can influence unfavorably the patient's response to measures ordinarily used in the treatment of congestive heart failure. Disturbances in the electrolyte balance may threaten the life of the individual in a number of other ways. For example, either extreme in potassium balance, namely potassium intoxication or potassium depletion, can paralyze skeletal muscle and, much more importantly, cardiac muscle. Though the condition which leads to the electrolyte imbalance may be a perfectly reversible and self-limited one, the very imbalance itself, unless recognized and corrected, can, through this cardiac effect, prove fatal. Electrolyte imbalance can imperil the individual not only through this direct effect, but through its effect in potentiating or initiating the toxic effect of certain pharmacologic agents. Thus in a patient receiving maintenance and hitherto non-toxic doses of digitalis, the loss of potassium from the body can precipitate digitalis poisoning; the loss of potassium is equivalent to giving the patient further increments of digitalis.[1]

POTASSIUM INTOXICATION

Potassium intoxication may result from excessive catabolism or administration or from inadequate excretion of this element, but generally, if not always, transient or permanent renal impairment is a prerequisite to the development of potassium intoxication. It can develop chronically or terminally in chronic renal disease with uremia. It can also appear rapidly in acute renal failure as a result of a number of causes. This includes carbon tetrachloride poisoning, acute tubular necrosis, the so-called "lower nephron syndrome" and the precipitation of sulfonamide crystals in the renal tubules. Here the defect is the decreased excretion of potassium liberated by the various normal catabolic processes. Potassium intoxication may also be due to acute hemolytic crises or the absorption of extravasated blood in the bowel or elsewhere. Any hemolytic process can predispose to potassium intoxication because of the liberation of potassium. It may also develop following the transfusion of incompatible blood. Here the two mechanisms are combined, excessive liberation of potassium from the breakdown of red cells and deficient excretion due to tubular necrosis. In the acute crisis of Addison's disease or in acute diabetic acidosis, potassium intoxication may be associated with hyponatremia. Here potassium intoxication arises as a consequence of faulty handling of potassium.

If, in any setting such as those just enumerated, the patient develops bradycardia, complains of a vague weakness or of loss of muscular strength, or develops a flaccid paralysis of the extremities, or even difficulty in phonation or respiration, potassium intoxication should be suspected. Sometimes the patient

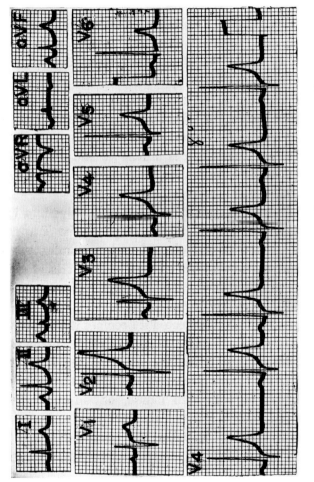

Fig. 11. *Potassium Intoxication in Acute Addisonian Crisis.* Note tall, narrow and peaked T waves. Though potassium intoxication is a regular feature of adrenal crisis, tracings of this type are rarely recorded. Clinicians wisely prefer to proceed with the management of the emergency rather than have an electrocardiogram taken at this juncture.

becomes semi-stuporous or lapses into a deep coma. Sometimes he complains of a burning sensation in the soles of his feet. The suspicion may be confirmed by the symmetrical diminution or absence of deep tendon or superficial cutaneous reflexes. Frequently the patient remains alert though apprehensive even after the reflexes have disappeared. The diagnosis should be confirmed by the electrocardiogram. Generally diagnostic electrocardiographic changes will have been present long before any of these clinical appearances have manifested themselves. The most available and reliable tool for detecting potassium intoxication is the direct recording electrocardiogram.[2] The estimation of the serum potassium level is time-consuming and therefore delayed; it is unreliable and undecisive for it does not furnish as complete information as does the electrocardiogram.

The earliest electrocardiographic evidence of potassium intoxication consists of a change in the shape of the T wave which becomes peaked or tent-shaped and, generally, symmetrical, tall and narrow. (Figs. 11 and 12,A) It is at this stage of T wave peaking that potassium intoxication must be recognized for the threat that it represents to the patient's survival. Once this appearance is detected it becomes the responsibility of the attending physician to decide whether, on the one hand, the appearance is a static one and the result of some chronic condition such as chronic uremia or of the long-term administration of potassium iodide, or, on the other, whether this appearance is a transient phase in a progressive picture of advancing and potentially fatal potassium intoxication. Bearing in mind that the degree of intoxication can change very rapidly, even over the course of an hour, frequently repeated electrocardiograms are mandatory until it has been established that the patient is on an even electrolyte keel. Worsening is indicated by broadening and lowering of the P waves (intra-atrial block) (Fig. 12, B), lengthening of the P-R

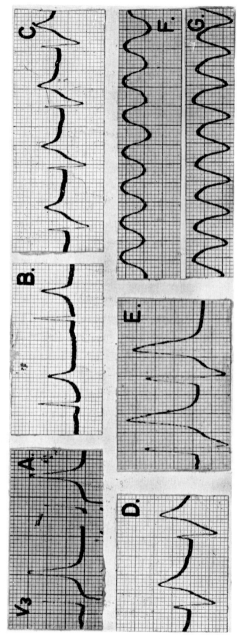

Fig. 12. *Spectrum of Electrocardiographic Changes in Potassium Intoxication.* With increasing severity of the process the pattern changes from one showing only T wave changes (A), through those showing lowered P waves (B), atrioventricular and intraventricular block (C and D), pronounced intraventricular block with atrial standstill (E), to ventricular flutter (F) or tachycardia (G).

interval (atrio-ventricular block) (Fig. 12, C) and widening of the QRS complex (intraventricular block) (Figs. 12, C, D and E) developing more or less concurrently. The latter is generally a diffuse affair but may transiently assume the appearance of right or left bundle branch block. As the degree of poisoning progresses, P waves are no longer recognizable (atrial standstill) and the ventricular complexes lose their angularity and become rounded off, eventually assuming a constant or variable sinuous (Fig. 12, F) or undulatory (Fig. 12, G) appearance (ventricular "flutter" or tachycardia), giving way terminally to erratic fine oscillations (ventricular fibrillation) or total quiescence (ventricular standstill) of the baseline. There is some variability in the order of these changes. This electrocardiographic spectrum parallels changes in the serum potassium value but it must be emphasized that the correlation is only an approximate one, and is probably influenced by the interplay of other serum electrolytes. Thus, at a given serum potassium level, a lowering of the serum sodium level induces a more profound electrocardiographic effect than a normal serum sodium level. Similarly a lowering of the serum calcium level enhances the electrocardiographic effect of a given serum potassium value while with a normal calcium a less pronounced electrocardiographic effect is recorded. Increasing acidosis may likewise accentuate potassium intoxication. It appears that the electrocardiogram is the composite effect of a number of variables in the serum and in the cell and that it faithfully reflects the totality of these effects at the myocardial cell membrane. It is this effect which is a much more reliable clue to clinical danger than is any single chemical determination such as the serum potassium level. Over the years, with one or two possible exceptions, the electrocardiogram has remained a reliable indicator of potassium intoxication.

The treatment of potassium intoxication is approached in two ways, in the long run through correction of the underlying cause, if correctable, and immediately through emergency measures designed to lower the serum potassium level. In many cases the cause of potassium intoxication is a self-limited one from which the patient may be expected to recover spontaneously, assuming that he can be tided over the emergency of possible cardiac arrest. If the patient is on potassium therapy, this should, of course, be stopped at once; I have seen cases in which it had been intended that potassium therapy be stopped weeks previously but where, through an error, this oral order had never been transmitted to the order book. If the condition is mild and stationary, it may be necessary to do nothing more than await the spontaneous clearing of its cause. In rapidly progressive potassium intoxication it is mandatory that the serum potassium level be lowered to or toward normal. Certain forms of therapy are rapid in their effect; these are likewise rapid in losing their effect. Others are slow in onset but persistent in maintaining their effect. If an immediate lowering of potassium is indicated one may infuse hypertonic sodium bicarbonate solution. Sodium ion antagonizes potassium effect and alkaline solutions lower serum potassium. Three ampoules of sodium bicarbonate, each containing 44 milliequivalents of sodium ion, are made up to 500 cc. This totals 132 milliequivalents of sodium. Somewhat less useful but a little more rapidly effective if the patient is hypocalcemic is calcium gluconate. This may be given undiluted as 1 gram in a 10 cc. ampoule or it may be diluted, giving, say, 2 grams in 100 cc. of 5% glucose solution. Somewhat slower but more persistent is glucose with insulin. This combination is useful for "follow-up" therapy. One may give 50 to 75 grams of glucose and 25 to 35 units of insulin (generally one unit of crystalline-zinc-insulin to 2 grams of glucose) in a 20 to 25% solution over the course of an hour in whatever volume it is felt that the patient can tolerate.[2] Sodium lactate may be used instead of bicarbonate. The lactate ion has to be metabolized;

[161]

this presumably accounts for the slight delay in its effect. Since this comes commercially as molar sodium lactate in a 100 cc. ampoule, it must be diluted. One must calculate how many milliequivalents of sodium are in the ampoule, make up as much of this solution as contains 150 milliequivalents and infuse this in 500 cc. of glucose in water. In other words it is given in the same strength as the bicarbonate solution. Sodium chloride may accomplish the same purpose but it is an acid salt. Acidosis tends to draw potassium out of the cells; the excess chloride ion counteracts the effect of sodium in antagonizing potassium. The end result may be little or no lowering of the serum potassium level. Bicarbonate solution is therefore preferred.

If 24 hours or more are available in which to combat potassium intoxication, a combination of Sorbitol and the exchange resin, Kay-exalate, may prove effective. Sorbitol is a poly-alcohol which is only partly absorbed. One gives 30 cc. by mouth. This keeps bowel contents moving along. If the patient has moderate potassium intoxication one then gives 15 grams of Kay-exalate. This exchanges sodium for potassium and binds potassium in the bowel. The resin may solidify in the bowel if rapid diarrhoea is not continued. If this material must be tube-fed a rubber, rather than a plastic, tube should be used. Once the potassium level has been lowered the resin is continued in a dose of 5 grams three or four times daily with enough Sorbitol to induce two bowel movements daily. This extremely effective form of therapy may be used if there is no contraindication to producing diarrhoea. Its use may even lead to potassium depletion and, if the patient has been receiving digitalis, to digitalis intoxication.

Alternately potassium may be extracted from the body by dialysis. "Artificial kidneys," now generally available in metropolitan and teaching centers, require skilled personnel working together as teams. The procedure is elaborate and costly but in certain cases where other measures have failed or been only partially or briefly effective, it may prove lifesaving. Tremendous amounts of potassium may also be removed by the alternative process of transperitoneal dialysis. This procedure is useful where the degree of heparinization necessary for hemodialysis with the artificial kidney is contraindicated. It is more generally available for it employs inexpensive and simple materials and basic techniques which are at hand in a community hospital.[3] The necessary apparatus consists of an ordinary intravenous infusion set, a routine paracentesis set containing a trocar with two stylets, one sharp, 15 to 20 cms. in length and with an outside diameter of 2.5 mms., the other blunt (the ordinary perforated hollow stylet commonly used for paracentesis), and two 30 cm. polyvinyl catheters which can be inserted through the trocar. Eight to 10 small smooth holes are made near the distal parts of the catheters which are hardened by immersion in mineral oil which has been heated almost to the boiling point (350°) and which can be autoclaved. Two plastic or metal adapters connect the catheter with the intravenous infusion apparatus. An irrigating fluid is now commercially available under the name of Peridial with 1½% glucose (Cutter) in one liter flasks. For patients with marked edema Peridial is available with 7% glucose to be used during the first few exchanges.

Just before the dialysis is started 100,000 units of penicillin, 50 mgms. of streptomycin and 5 mgms. of heparin are added. A flat film is taken of the abdomen to observe possible filling of the bowel with gas or feces. The patient is sedated and given a gentle enema. With the patient on his back in a comfortable position and his head and shoulders supported on a pillow, the skin of the abdomen is prepared as if for a laparotomy, small wheals are raised with 1 or 2% procaine, one at about McBurney's point and the other at a corresponding position on the left. A small incision is made on the left-sided wheal and the trocar, with the sharp stylet in place, is inserted through the subcutaneous tissues and, with a sharp thrust, through the aponeurosis of the external oblique muscle. The sharp stylet is now replaced by the blunt stylet and the peritoneum entered with another vigorous thrust. The plastic catheter is inserted through the trocar for a distance of 10 to 20 cms., the metal trocar removed, the catheter connected to the intravenous set containing the bottle of irrigating fluid with plastic or metal adapters, the catheter fixed to the abdominal wall and the paracentesis site draped with a sterile towel. Fluid, warmed to body temperature, is allowed to flow in from 2-liter flasks at the rate of 2 liters per hour. After running about ¾ hour, when the abdomen is obviously distended, the outflow catheter is similarly inserted and connected to a collecting flask beneath the patient's bed. To avoid excessive distention and consequent pain the rate of inflow should be adjusted to that of outflow. A constant volume of about 2 liters is maintained in the peritoneal cavity. In general the rate of inflow is maintained at 2 to 3 liters per hour for 12 to 15 hours. A longer dialysis is apt to induce infection. At the end of the procedure both catheters are removed. A residual of 1000 to 1500 cc. is inevitable and must be taken into consideration in estimating subsequent fluid requirements. The dialysis may be repeated in 48 hours.

Each and all of the procedures enumerated are monitored constantly with the electrocardiogram. Treatment is adequate and may be omitted, temporarily at least, when the tracing again shows a normal morphology or the baseline appearance which antedated the development of potassium intoxication. Appropriate therapy may be resumed on its redevelopment.

POTASSIUM DEPLETION

In general hospital practice potassium depletion is about five times as frequent as potassium intoxication. It may come about as a result of excessive elimination or inadequate intake of potassium or of abnormal transfers of the element.[4] It may result from the loss of potassium in body fluids through vomiting or diarrhoea, by nasogastric suction, intestinal intubation, or from gastrointestinal fistulae, through large abdominal paracenteses, through copious mercurial or Diuril-induced diureses, in so-called "potassium-losing" nephritis or during the infusion of fluids deficient in potassium. It may likewise be a clue to hyperaldosteronism. Potassium depletion is frequently associated with alkalosis and with a lowered extracellular or serum potassium. A fall in serum potassium may also be effected by a redistribution of potassium between the intra- and extra-cellular compartments. This can occur in the crises of familial or acquired periodic paralysis, in Addison's disease being treated with desoxycorticosterone acetate, during the correction of diabetic acidosis as a consequence of the insulin-induced transport of potassium from serum to cells when supplemental potassium is not given, or following the rapid overcorrection of potassium intoxication. I have seen the same sort of reversal from potassium intoxication to potassium depletion after a brisk spontaneous diuresis following renal shut-down. During the first few days after surgery, particularly cardiac surgery, there is a dilution hyponatremia and the urinary potassium excretion increases. This is paralleled by a rise in the serum potassium level and fall in the serum sodium level. This phenomenon, which is maximal on the second post-operative day, corresponds to the time of maximal diuresis and the maximal incidence of atrial fibrillation. It generally rectifies itself in the next few days.

Clinically potassium depletion should be suspected when the extremities become weak or paralyzed, when the patient becomes hoarse or aphonic or when he develops ileus. When these conditions are present potassium depletion is extreme and verification easy. Lesser degrees of depletion should be suspected merely on the basis of a clinical setting appropriate for their development. The confirmation of partial depletion is much more difficult. It is important to bear in mind the distinction between total body potassium depletion, and lowering of the serum potassium level (hypokalemia or hypopotassemia). It is not clear yet which of these factors determines clinical or electrocardiographic phenomena or whether these are perhaps determined by simple or complex interrelationships between these factors. In the present state of our ignorance it is therefore better to refer to this condition as potassium depletion.

The electrocardiogram generally shows characteristic changes when the degree of depletion is great. With mild to moderate losses of potassium from the body the electrocardiogram is frequently helpful; at this stage it may well furnish the first clue to its development. The electrocardiogram may show a whole spectrum of changes some of which are merely compatible with, some of which are quite suggestive of, or even distinctive of, potassium depletion, but there is no single electrocardiographic feature which is pathognomonic. It is frequently difficult to distinguish the changes of potassium depletion from those due to the absorption of quinidine or digitalis or to myocardial ischemia. The changes consist of lowering (Fig. 13,A,E and F), notching (Fig. 13,C and D) or flattening (Fig. 13,B,F and G) of the T wave, depression of the RS-T segments (Fig. 13,E,F and G), prolongation of the Q-T interval (Fig. 13,C and G) and the development or augmentation of a U wave (Fig. 13,B,C,D,E,F,G and H) which becomes prominent relative to the T wave. The changes may proceed singly or in combination. When the changes are combined and the tracings show depressed RS-T segments, inverted T waves and prominent U waves (Fig. 13,F and G), they may be considered quite distinctive. With time one observes a dynamic amoeboid growth of the U wave at the expense of the T wave. The notching of the T waves when

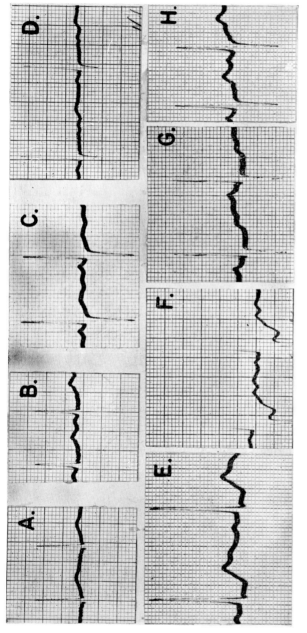

Fig. 13. *Panorama of Electrocardiographic Changes in Potassium Depletion.* Lowering of T wave (A), prominence of U wave (B), notching of T wave (C), triple contour of T-U sector (D), depression of RS-T segment with prominent U wave and T larger than U (E), same with T equalling U (F), same with U larger than T (G), and one with flat T but prominent U (H). The changes resemble those induced by quinidine, except that potassium depletion does not cause intraventricular block

combined with a prominent U wave imparts a characteristic rolling triple-notched contour to the T and U sector of the electrocardiogram (Fig. 13,C and D). In a number of cases the P-R interval may be prolonged and the P waves prominent. Atrioventricular nodal rhythm is not uncommon. Many arrhythmias, supraventricular and ventricular, may be precipitated during the loss of potassium, especially when this is a rapid loss, whether or not the patient has been receiving digitalis, but it is principally the digitalis-induced arrhythmias which are triggered when the body is depleted of potassium. This includes ventricular or supraventricular premature beats, atrioventricular block or dissociation and ventricular or supraventricular tachycardia, notably atrial tachycardia with block.

Potassium depletion may also be reflected in a lowering of the serum potassium below the normal range of 3.8 to 5.0 milliequivalents per liter. But the serum potassium level may remain within the normal range when the body is depleted of small to moderate amounts of potassium. In the presence of acidosis potassium depletion may be present in spite of a normal or even slightly elevated serum potassium level. There is frequently a plateau below which the serum potassium is not readily lowered; further losses of body potassium may have little or no effect upon the serum potassium level and presumably are derived from within the cells. When the degree of potassium depletion is slight, then, either the electrocardiogram or the serum potassium level may be within normal limits.[5] At this stage the electrocardiogram may suggest potassium depletion while the serum potassium is normal; or conversely the serum potassium level may be depressed when the electrocardiogram is within normal limits. The use of both of these parameters will therefore pick up more instances of potassium depletion than either alone. When the degree of potassium depletion is considerable, each, the electrocardiogram and the serum potassium level, is likely to be abnormal. At times I have seen a lag of a day or two before total body potassium loss or repletion is reflected in the electrocardiogram or in the serum potassium level.

Potassium depletion is treated by elimination or control of its cause, if feasible, and, more importantly, by replacement of body stores with potassium. Thus diuretic measures should be discontinued or suspended, appropriate anti-diarrhoeal measures instituted and abdominal paracenteses avoided. Frequently it is necessary to continue the very measures, such as nasogastric suction, which are known certainly or possibly to underlie the depletion. Depending upon the clinical situation potassium may be given orally or intravenously. Where the patient's condition is not critical, it may be given by mouth in the form of 1 gram enteric coated tablets of potassium chloride, as solution of Potassium Triplex or as Elixir Kaon* (potassium gluconate). The initial dose might be 3 grams, repeated one and two hours later if necessary. Where a more rapid effect seems desirable, 5 grams (67 milliequivalents) may be given in a glass of iced orange juice. In milder cases one simply gives one gram three times daily over a number of days. The disadvantages of oral medication are that one may overshoot the mark, inducing potassium intoxication, and that the administered dose cannot be retrieved. If the condition of the patient seems more urgent, or if he has renal disease, intravenous infusion is undertaken with constant electrocardiographic monitoring, discontinuing the infusion immediately the T waves become peaked. In those cases in which potassium is given in this manner for an arrhythmia or other toxic effect of digitalis, the infusion is stopped upon the disappearance of the arrhythmia or other toxic manifestation if this occurs before the T waves become tented. For intravenous therapy 3 grams (40 milliequivalents) of potassium are given in 500 cc. of 5% glucose in water over the course of an hour. One must be par-

* 15 cc. = 20 mEq.

ticularly cautious in the use of potassium in elderly individuals, in patients in congestive heart failure and those with chronic renal disease.

REFERENCES

(1) Lown, B. and Levine, H. D.: Atrial Arrhythmias, Digitalis and Potassium. Landsberger Medical Books, Inc., New York, 1958.
(2) Merrill, J. P., Levine, H. D., Somerville, W. and Smith, S., 3rd.: Clinical recognition and treatment of acute potassium intoxication. Ann. Int. Med. 33: 797, 1950.
(3) Legrain, M. and Merrill, J. P.: Short-term continuous transperitoneal dialysis. N.E.J. Med. 248: 125, 1953.
(4) Levine, H. D.: Electrolyte imbalance and the electrocardiogram. Modern Concepts of Cardiovascular Disease. 23: 246, 1954.
(5) Schwartz, W. B., Levine, H. D. and Relman, A. S.: The electrocardiogram in potassium depletion. Its relation to the total potassium deficit and the serum concentration. Am. J. Med. 16: 395, 1954.

8

DIGITALIS INTOXICATION

Subjective Manifestations

Arrhythmias

Treatment

8

DIGITALIS INTOXICATION

The digitalis glycosides, after nearly 200 years of continuous use, are still among the most useful drugs in the treatment of heart disease. This despite the narrow margin between therapeutic and toxic dosage. It has generally been agreed that over the past two decades there has been a definite increase in the incidence of poisoning induced by these glycosides. This increase is in part attributable to the more widespread use of the drug and in part to the fact that people with heart disease live longer and therefore have more advanced heart disease than was the case a generation ago. When a patient has received a therapeutic dose of digitalis he has already received 60% of the potentially toxic dose. This is true, no matter which preparation is used, whether it be crude digitalis leaf or any one of the purified glycosides. With advancing age of the patient or with a greater severity of the underlying heart disease, this therapeutic-toxic ratio narrows.[1] It is very difficult to produce fatal poisoning with digitalis if the heart is normal.[2,3] Massive doses, even as large as 50 mgms. of Digitaline Nativelle, have been consumed at one time without fatality when the heart was normal.

It was one of the teachings of Dr. Henry Christian, who had a tremendous influence in the promotion of digitalis therapy in this country, that the drug should be given to the point of minor toxic symptoms such as anorexia or nausea. At this juncture he advised omitting the drug for 48 hours or so, with resumption of maintenance doses thereafter. The onset merely of subjective evidence of toxicity may herald the imminence of grave arrhythmias. Because of this, some physicians attempt to stop short of these minor toxic symptoms; but this is often difficult to gauge. Dr. Christian also emphasized that the digitalizing and maintenance requirements must be determined for each patient by the process of trial and error. Experience with the purified glycosides re-emphasizes the lesson that each digitalization must be regarded as an individual titration. Ready-made dosage schedules have only statistical meaning and are of no value in predicting the requirements of the individual patient. It should be clear that this very method of digitalization, to which most of us subscribe, necessarily entails, for a time at least, minor degrees of digitalis intoxication.

Toxicity is much more likely to develop in patients with coexistent kidney or liver disease, be it primary liver impairment or such hepatic changes as chronic passive congestion or "cardiac cirrhosis." This is because digitalis is excreted in the kidney, detoxified in the liver. We haven't much information beyond clinical impression that faulty renal function and resultant failure of excretion of the drug can contribute to toxicity. But the effect of liver disease upon digitalis requirement is well illustrated in the experimental observations of Lown who found, in the dog whose portal vein was cannulated, that 3 or 4 times the same dose of acetylstrophanthidin is required to produce an end-point of ventricular tachycardia when the drug is injected into the portal vein than when it is injected directly into a systemic vein which by-passes the liver.[4]

With advancing age, more severe heart disease or more pronounced degrees of congestive heart failure, or any combination of these factors, it may be difficult or impossible to achieve a beneficial effect of the drug without some toxic symptoms. And there are probably some rare individuals who show symptoms of digitalis poisoning even before a therapeutic effect is attained.[3]

A final factor, perhaps the most important of all, which has contributed to the increasing incidence of digitalis intoxication, is the procedures currently used in the management of congestive heart failure. This includes reliance upon electrolyte manipulations, such as restriction in salt intake, the use of such diuretic agents as the mercurial drugs, Diamox, Diuril, ammonium chloride, the mechanical removal of serous effusions by chest or belly taps or the use of Southey's tubes and the employment of steroids. These procedures, as successful as they may be and have been in the treatment of cardiac decompensation, alone or in concert have the common tendency of depleting the body of potassium. Although other electrolyte changes may be of some importance in precipitating digitalis intoxication, it is probable that potassium is the key ion.[1] Other factors possibly inducing potassium loss and thus affecting the digitalis-potassium relationship are described in the preceding chapter. There is good reason to believe that the very process of congestive heart failure and that the drug, digitalis, each is capable of bringing about a loss of bodily, and specifically of cellular, potassium. This applies to the tissues in general and the heart in particular. Progressive loss of potassium sensitizes the heart to the toxic action of digitalis. The physician must expect, therefore, that either or both of these factors may underlie his patient's toxicity.

Before proceeding to a consideration of the various manifestations of digitalis intoxication, two common errors deserve correction. These are the practice of treating a rapid heart, merely because it is rapid, with digitalis, and that of assessing the adequacy of digitalis therapy by its effect upon the ventricular complex of the electrocardiogram.

Sinus tachycardia should not be treated with digitalis. This is generally a compensatory mechanism. Other things being equal, the more rapid rate makes for an increased output of the heart. Even where curtailed diastole decreases the stroke volume output, up to a certain point the increased rate may overbalance this effect, resulting in an increased minute volume output of the heart. Giving digitalis under these circumstances can be dangerous. The treatment of sinus tachycardia is the treatment of its cause.

Digitalis may induce a cupped-depressed or hammock-shaped or sagging contour of the RS-T segment, a shortening of the Q-T interval and inversion of the T waves. These effects indicate neither adequacy of digitalis dosage nor a toxic effect of digitalis. It is hazardous and unjustified therefore to try to gauge adequacy of digitalis dosage from the electrocardiogram. They do suggest absorption of the drug. The digitalis deformity bears some resemblance to that induced by subendocardial ischemia or potassium depletion; in rare instances it is impossible to make the distinction. In the patient presenting this electrocardiographic feature, who denies having received the drug, renewed and careful inquiry is mandatory regarding so-called "tonics" or proprietary preparations, one of whose ingredients, like the brew of the old lady of Shropshire, might be digitalis.

SUBJECTIVE MANIFESTATIONS

Gastrointestinal Symptoms Probably the best known toxic symptoms induced by overdosage of digitalis are gastrointestinal in origin. This includes anorexia, nausea, vomiting and diarrhoea. It is generally considered that these are due to the central effects of the digitalis bodies themselves, located either in the heart or the brain. These effects can be induced by each and every one of the digitalis preparations. It is true that the non-absorbed moiety of the crude preparations can induce nausea or vomiting by virtue of a local effect upon the gastrointestinal mucosa, an effect that is generally less pronounced with the purified derivatives. Yet it is probable that those of us who were brought up in the digitalis leaf era used this end point successfully as an effective guide to digitalis toxicity. Because digitalization may be more rapidly achieved with the purified drugs, their first effects may be arrhythmic rather than gastrointestinal. The proponents of the use of the purified preparations argue that some of the gastrointestinal symptoms are produced by impurities and not by the active principles of digitalis, that they need not be a true and reliable guide to toxicity and that the same margin between therapeutic and toxic doses exists with regard to all preparations. For the present the physician will continue to use that digitalis preparation with which he is familiar. It is important to recognize that these very gastrointestinal symptoms may be the effect not of digitalis but of the process of cardiac decompensation and the resultant congestion of the gastrointestinal tract and liver. In such an instance their development may be an indication for initiating, re-initiating, continuing or increasing digitalis rather than a contraindication to its further use.

I have seen a number of patients on maintenance digitalis therapy who lost their appetites and slowly lost large amounts of weight over long periods of time. They were suspected of having developed carcinoma and were studied extensively and expensively. Cancer was not found. Excepting anorexia they presented no other evidence suggesting digitalis intoxication. Yet in each case omission of digitalis until the appetite returned, and the subsequent resumption of the drug in smaller dosage was followed by progressive return to the previous weight. The anorectic effect of digitalis may develop, then, during maintenance therapy as well as during initial digitalization.

Central Nervous System Symptoms Colored vision was de-

scribed in the classic publication on digitalis therapy of Withering,[5] and has been described by many others, yet there are
many physicians who claim that they have never observed this
phenomenon. The point is well made by Sprague, White and
Kellogg [6] that one must inquire specifically regarding this
symptom, else it be missed. The patient may complain of diffuse
yellow, green or orange vision or of the presence of colored dots
floating by. Sometimes the complaint is of silvery streaks
streaming across the field of vision.

Such mental symptoms as confusion and delirium are commonly ignored as manifestations of digitalis intoxication and
are attributed rather to a "cardiac psychosis." The possible confusion of these symptoms with those of ammonium intoxication
has been discussed on page 144. While ammonium intoxication
carries a grave prognosis, this may not be the case with recognized digitalis intoxication.

There is some evidence that digitalis may increase the sensitivity of the carotid sinus.[7] It has been suggested that individuals who have had asymptomatic carotid sinus sensitivity before
receiving digitalis may first develop syncope only after being
digitalized.

Muscular Weakness Muscular weakness is a little known
toxic effect of digitalis. LaDue [8] described the development of
cramps, weakness and heaviness in the muscles as well as di-
plopia in a girl receiving increments of digitalis. Prompted by
this single clinical experience he found that digitalis induced
progressive muscular weakness and diminished or abolished the
ability of dogs to exercise on a treadmill. It seems quite possible that this weakness is related to muscular potassium deficiency induced by digitalis.

Miscellaneous True sensitivity to digitalis in the sense that
the drug cannot be tolerated at all because of the presence of
an allergy to the drug or the production by it of blood dyscra-
sia or the like just does not exist. At least I know of no proven

instance of such sensitivity and have never observed one personally. Sensitivity in the sense of an extraordinarily small requirement of the drug for digitalization or maintenance does exist. There are some individuals, for example, who develop toxic symptoms as a result of the administration of doses which in other individuals would be considered small maintenance doses.[3] Generally speaking, alleged instances of sensitivity are the result of improper coaching of the patient by the physician initiating digitalis therapy. If it has been made clear from the outset that the development of minor toxic symptoms are a signal merely for temporary omission rather than total suspension of the drug, the number of such instances will be reduced.

Gynecomastia is a rare but disturbing toxic effect of chronic digitalis administration. Hyperpigmentation of the areolae, on the other hand, is a very common effect of digitalis. It is doubtful, however, that this should be regarded as a toxic phenomenon; this finding, which has been explained on the basis of the structural similarity of digitalis to the steroids, is certainly no contraindication to proceeding with the drug.

ARRHYTHMIAS

There is no toxic rhythm which cannot, at some time or other, be induced by digitalis. The simplest and most familiar of these is ventricular premature beats. It is recognized, of course, that this arrhythmia may be a manifestation not of digitalis overdosage but of the process of congestive heart failure and thus actually constitute an indication for digitalis therapy. If the ventricular premature beats vary in form they are much more likely to be the result of digitalis intoxication.

Ventricular Premature Beats Versus Aberrant Ventricular Conduction

The detection of true ventricular premature beats in patients with atrial fibrillation should make one hesitate to give further increments of digitalis. But all abnormal looking ventricular complexes developing during atrial fibrillation are not necessarily ventricular premature beats; some of them may be the result of aberrant ventricular spread of beats which actually arise in the atria. This form of aberrant ventricular conduction is predicated upon the so-called "Ashman phenomenon" which is conditioned by the effect of cycle length upon refractory period. With a normal sinus mechanism the refractory period is prolonged when the heart rate is slow and cycle length long; the refractory period is short when the heart rate is rapid and cycle length short. This relationship also holds in hearts with atrial fibrillation but because of the variation in cycle length and a possible lag in these relationships, the refractory period of a given beat may not be so easy to estimate. It may be stated as a general proposition, however, that in atrial fibrillation the refractory period of a given beat is determined by the pause which just precedes that beat. If the pause is short, the refractory period of the succeeding beat is short; if the pause is long, the succeeding refractory period is long. But the refractory period is not identical in all units of the ventricular myocardium; there is an interval in the latter part of the refractory period of the ventricle as a whole when some of the fibers have recovered their responsiveness and others have not. After a long pause an impulse from the atria, which happens to reach the ventricular myocardium during this interval, will find some of the fibers responsive, others refractory; it will therefore pick a different course in the ventricles, resulting in a ventricular complex whose morphology is different from that of indigenous beats in the same lead. If, on the other hand, the preceding

[180]

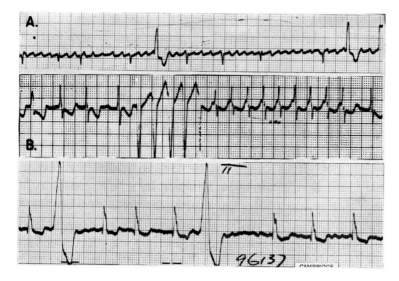

Fig. 14. *Aberrant Ventricular Conduction in Supraventricular Mechanisms.* (A) Aberrant ventricular beats in atrial fibrillation, developing shortly after ventricular beat preceded by a long pause. These beats generally show the configuration of complete or incomplete right bundle branch block, have no fixed time relationship to the preceding ventricular complex and are not followed by compensatory pauses. They do not contraindicate digitalis. (B) Repetitive aberration in atrial flutter in patient on quinidine therapy. The first aberrant beat is set up by a pause which is the longest in the lead. Following the five beats exhibiting aberration there is a 1:1 response with the ventricular complexes of normal duration. The rate is identical (215) during repetitive aberration and 1:1 response phase. Quinidine discontinued. (C) Ventricular premature beats during atrial fibrillation shown in contrast with (A) and (B). The pause preceding the beat which is followed by the abnormal beat is not unduly prolonged. The abnormal beat is followed by a "compensatory" pause.

[181]

cycle length is short, an impulse arriving at the ventricles from above at precisely the same instant would find all of the ventricular fibers responsive and a normal beat would result. In about 70% of cases the aberrantly conducted beat has the appearance of complete or incomplete right bundle branch block. Because the interval of partial responsiveness is not just one instant but has some, variable, duration, these aberrant beats have a varying relationship to the preceding ventricular complex; true ventricular premature beats, on the other hand, are quite fixed in their timing following the previous beat. Another helpful differentiating point is that with aberrant ventricular conduction the abnormal beat is not followed by a compensatory pause whereas a true ventricular premature beat, even in atrial fibrillation, tends to be followed by a "compensatory" or compensatory-like pause; the ventricular premature beat tends to penetrate the atrio-ventricular conduction pathway by retrograde conduction so that beats which happen subsequently to filter down from the atria find the conduction pathway to be refractory for some time. This does not occur when the beats are conducted in a normal forward direction from auricle to ventricle. Bearing these considerations in mind, one can generally differentiate between ventricular premature beats and aberrant ventricular conduction. Aberrant ventricular conduction is not a contraindication to proceeding with digitalis. There are some patients whose electrocardiograms, when examined from this standpoint, show both aberrant ventricular conduction and ventricular premature beats. In this dilemma the decision whether digitalis therapy should be continued must depend upon other factors.

Bigeminal rhythm does not result from the aberrant ventricular conduction which is thus induced. Bigeminal rhythm, or coupling, may be due to ventricular premature beats. But there is an entire catalogue of other mechanisms which can induce bigeminy.[9] Included in this group are certain disorders of impulse formation (sinus bigeminy, ventricular parasystole) and disorders of impulse conduction, alone or in combination. Among the more common arrhythmias in the latter group are, with sinus rhythm, 3:2 A-V block and 3:2 S-A block; combinations of 2:1 and 3:2 conduction or alternations of 2:1 and 3:1 conduction in atrial flutter; reciprocal beating; and Wolff-Parkinson-White syndrome. All of these possibilities must be kept in mind and electrocardiograms recorded before the conclusion is drawn that the bigeminy is necessarily due to ventricular premature beats. Even when due to ventricular premature beats, bigeminal rhythm is not necessarily a manifestation of digitalis toxicity. In rheumatic heart disease such coupling is due to digitalis in 95% of cases, in coronary artery disease about 50%.[10] With underlying atrial fibrillation ventricular bigeminy is a toxic effect of digitalis most of the time, in normal sinus mechanism in about half of the cases. Although many people appear to do well in spite of a bigeminal rhythm for years, it is noteworthy that Corday has found a 25% reduction in cardiac output in bigeminy.[11,12] All other things being equal, therefore, a patient is better off with a normal mechanism. And, more important, until one knows otherwise, his bigeminy may be the precursor of a more advanced and dangerous arrhythmia. Therefore it is recommended that the digitalized cardiac be treated if he develops this arrhythmia. It is worth remembering also that atrial premature beats may at times result from digitalis overdosage; I have seen them not infrequently as a harbinger of atrial tachycardia with block.

Let us imagine that you are in the process of treating a patient with atrial fibrillation with increments of digitalis. At evening rounds you find her apical rate to be 110 and the rhythm grossly irregular. On the following morning you find the rhythm regular, the rate, say, 100. Your normal impulse now will be to attribute this change to reversion to normal sinus rhythm. And let it be said here that though pharmacolo-

[183]

gists say that digitalis tends to perpetuate rather than terminate atrial fibrillation, reversion to a normal mechanism occurs under digitalis therapy much more often than the text books would lead us to expect. But, if you go to the trouble of taking an electrocardiogram at this point, you may find that the ventricles are indeed regular, but that the auricles continue to fibrillate. This is then not a sinus mechanism but nodal tachycardia which is a toxic digitalis effect. If this were not recognized and digitalis therapy continued, the rate of the nodal tachycardia would become faster. In the face of a rising heart rate the tendency is to give more and more digitalis. The result can well be fatal digitalis intoxication. There are two important lessons to be learned from such an experience, namely, that the sudden regularization of a previously irregular rhythm may mean not restoration of a normal rhythm but the development of digitalis toxicity. The progressive increase in the heart rate has similar implications. This does not mean that all patients whose heart rates accelerate while receiving digitalis are receiving toxic doses of the drug. In some of them the underlying condition is worsening or they have developed some complication: these probably need more digitalis. But the possibility of digitalis poisoning must be considered.

Tachycardia of the node can also develop when the auricles are still beating regularly. The atrioventricular node may eventually attain a rate which is faster than that of the atria. This is the hallmark of atrioventricular dissociation. This term once was used synonymously with atrioventricular block. Nowadays it has acquired a quite different meaning. Atrioventricular block implies a delay in the passage of the impulse from auricles to ventricles or a barrier to that passage so that one or more beats do not reach the ventricles. Atrioventricular dissociation, on the contrary, indicates an enhancement or whipping up in the automaticity of the atrioventricular node so that the ventricle constantly or periodically beats faster than the atrium. The ventricle, as it were, "gets its punches in quicker" than the auricle. Conduction is still possible between auricles and ventricles; if a beat of atrial origin happens to present at the atrioventricular node at an opportune moment it will be conducted. This we now call a ventricular capture. Some people call this "interference with dissociation" but this term has so many different meanings to so many different authorities that it is perhaps best discarded. Those cases of dissociation in which none of the auricular beats are conducted through to the ventricles will be called complete atrioventricular dissociation, those in which there is an occasional ventricular capture will be called partial atrioventricular dissociation. Any of these mechanisms can develop as a consequence of excessive doses of digitalis.

Ventricular tachycardia and fibrillation can also be due to digitalis intoxication. In fact digitalis bio-assay methods depend upon an endpoint of ventricular fibrillation, going through the sequence of ventricular premature beats, ventricular tachycardia and ventricular fibrillation. The lesser toxic rhythms described in this chapter are significant principally in that they are to be regarded as way-stations along the road to fatal ventricular fibrillation. The management of ventricular tachycardia and fibrillation is described in Chapters 13 and 14. Bidirectional ventricular tachycardia is practically pathognomonic of digitalis intoxication. This condition is discussed further on page 276. Atrial tachycardia with block is due to digitalis intoxication in about 70% of cases. This disturbance is discussed fully in Chapter 11.

TREATMENT

Digitalis toxicity is treated first of all by omitting digitalis. Among the factors which influence the duration of toxicity after stopping the drug are the severity of the underyling heart disease, the duration of overdosage and the particular digitalis preparation employed. Digitoxin is generally excreted by 1–3 weeks, digoxin by 1–3 days and ouabain in a matter of hours. Generally the toxic effect will have disappeared by the end of two weeks but it may last over a month. Frequently this is all that needs to be done. It is probably wise to omit all diuretic measures at the same time, certainly if a large diuresis occurred at about or just before the time of the development of toxicity. From this point on the least that one can do, in addition, is not to disturb the electrolyte balance unfavorably. Depending upon one's estimate of the gravity of the situation, potassium will be supplemented. This is discussed in detail on page 169.

Patients with chronic congestive heart failure handle potassium poorly and are prone to develop potassium intoxication on doses of potassium which are ordinarily regarded as harmless. Digitalis is not commonly given in the absence of cardiac decompensation. The group of patients being discussed in this chapter is therefore vulnerable to potassium intoxication. Hence either against an anticipated toxic rhythm or upon the disappearance of known arrhythmia, a blanket policy of constant prophylactic potassium therapy is not justified. The decision whether potassium should be instituted or continued must depend upon the actual or anticipated experience of the patient with regard to this cation. On the other hand the use of small doses of potassium, namely less than 1 gram a day, is merely an amulet which affords no protection.

Procaine amide is also effective against the arrhythmias due to digitalis intoxication. It will be the preferred medication in patients with renal insufficiency or potassium intoxication. But since this drug may significantly lower the blood pressure level, potassium will be preferred in hypotensive individuals. Procaine amide may be given by mouth in the dosage of 0.25 gram 4 i.d. or in progressively increasing dosage (0.25, 0.50, 0.75, 1.00 gram at 3 or 4 hour intervals). In more serious or desperate cases the drug may be given by vein in titrated increments of 50 mgms. (½ c.c.) every two minutes, pausing for electrocardiographic control and blood pressure determination before each addition. One may give up to 1000 or 2000 mgms. in this way. If the pressure falls the intervals are increased; if it then falls still lower the infusion is discontinued. This drug may also be given intramuscularly. The recommended initial dose is 0.5 to 2.0 grams followed by 0.5 to 1.0 gram at intervals determined by the response.

Chelating agents such as sodium ethylenediamine tetra-acetic acid (Na-EDTA) have also been recommended in digitalis intoxication.[13] The recommended dose is 600 mgms. given intravenously over the course of 15 to 30 minutes. My experience with this agent in these arrhythmias is too limited to justify an opinion on its value.

REFERENCES

(1) Lown, B. and Levine, S. A.: Current Concepts in Digitalis Therapy. Little, Brown and Co., Boston, Toronto, 1954.

(2) Duvoir, M., Pollet, L., Desoille, H. and Gaultier, M.: Deux cas d'intoxication par la digitaline. Étude electrocardiographique. Bull. et mém. Soc. méd. d. hôp. de Paris. 1: 159, 1938.

(3) Craig, L. C., Lown, B. and Levine, S. A.: Resistance and sensitivity to digitalis. J.A.M.A. 166: 2139, 1958.

(4) Lown, B., Whipple, G. H., Shoemaker, W. C., Craig, L. C. and Levine S. A.: Rôle of the liver in digitalis-induced electrolyte shifts. Abstracts 31st Scientific Sessions, American Heart Ass'n. Circ. 18: 753, 1958.

(5) Withering, W.: An Account of the Foxglove and Some of its Medical Uses. Swinney, Birmingham, 1785.

(6) Sprague, H. B., White, P. D. and Kellogg, J. F.: Disturbances of vision due to digitalis. Review of the literature and report of cases. J.A.M.A. *85*: 716, 1925.

(7) Weiss, S., Capps, R. B., Ferris, E. B. and Munro, D.: Syncope and convulsion due to hyperactive carotid sinus reflex. Arch. Int. Med. *58*: 407, 1936.

(8) LaDue, J. S.: Generalized muscular weakness as a toxic reaction to digitalis. Proc. Soc. Exper. Biol. and Med. *48*: 5, 1941.

(9) Pick, A. and Langendorf, R.: Personal communication.

(10) Sagall, E. L. and Wolff, L.: Digitalis bigeminy: analysis of fifty cases. N.E.J. Med. *240*: 676, 1949.

(11) Corday, E., Gold, H., deVera, L. B., Williams, J. H. and Fields, J.: Effect of the cardiac arrhythmias on the coronary circulation. Ann. Int. Med. *50*: 535, 1959.

(12) Corday, E., Williams, J. H., deVera, L. B. and Gold, H.: Hemodynamics of the coronary circulation during cardiac arrhythmias. Modern Concepts Cardiovascular Disease. *27*: 493, 1958.

(13) Gubner, R. and Kallman, H.: Treatment of digitalis toxicity by chelation of serum calcium. Am. J. Med. Sci. *234*: 136, 1957.

CHAPTER

9

PAROXYSMAL ATRIAL

TACHYCARDIA

Diagnosis

Differential Diagnosis

Treatment

CHAPTER

9

PAROXYSMAL ATRIAL

TACHYCARDIA

Classical tachycardia of the auricles is generally so well recognized and well treated that it is much more frequently seen outside of than within hospital walls. This disturbance is abrupt in onset and offset. The rate of the heart generally varies between 140 and 240 beats per minute. Except during the first two or three and the last two or three beats of a paroxysm, the rhythm in an attack is generally perfectly regular. As a working rule, therefore, when the disturbance is established and persistent, the rhythm can be expected to be precisely regular. The attacks may last moments, hours, days or even weeks, but most of them are over within two or three hours. Many patients notice nothing more than a vague sense of uneasiness with their attacks and are able to continue about their usual duties. Most patients are quite aware of their attack. They suddenly feel a fast pounding in the chest and liken its regularity to that of a trip-hammer. Not so many are aware of its abrupt termination. Some actually have to be questioned as to its cessation. After a moment's reflection they may concede that it is now over. Some patients notice in addition to palpitation and tachycardia a sense of weariness, oppression or anxiety. Some notice true shortness of breath. Others describe their suffocation as an inability to, or a need to, take a satis-factory breath. Others, particularly those with coronary artery disease, are seized with substernal tightness or heaviness or pain. This may occur at the onset of an attack but is more likely to come on after it has lasted some time. Others describe a sense of gaseousness in the chest or epigastrium. I recall one patient who complained of attacks of "gas." Cholecystograms demonstrated gallstones. During the period following cholecys-tectomy she had another attack of "gas" identical with those she had before surgery. It was only then that I appreciated that her spells of "gas" were indeed bouts of atrial tachycardia.

In a few patients the symptoms may be so severe as to make the patient take to a chair or bed. There may be collapse, sweating, fever, leucocytosis and fall in blood pressure. In short, the attacks may be associated with many of the clinical and laboratory features of acute coronary thrombosis. Some individuals may faint at the onset of an attack. This symptom may also develop in other forms of paroxysmal rapid action of the heart (atrial flutter, atrial fibrillation, ventricular tachy-cardia). In investigating patients who have fainting attacks one must therefore always consider paroxysmal rapid heart action of any type.

The symptomatology is often profoundly affected by the previous experience of the patient with his attacks. The initial attack is very much an unknown quantity to the patient and is much more liable then to be regarded as an acute threat and therefore a medical emergency. After having been through a number of bouts the patient, particularly if he has had good medical advice, is more likely to take subsequent bouts in stride.

Paroxysmal atrial tachycardia may occur in the presence or absence of heart disease. In well over half of patients in my experience, the history, physical examination and thorough laboratory studies fail to reveal evidence of heart disease. In such patients a particular point should be made of reassuring them that they have no heart disease and that these attacks can occur when the heart is perfectly normal. Among those in whom organic heart disease is present, rheumatic, particularly mitral, thyrotoxic, hypertensive and coronary artery disease are the more common etiologic factors. Among the noncardiac organic etiologic causes of atrial tachycardia are alcohol, tobacco, acute infections, and acute allergic reactions but all of these are rare. The chief clinical importance of the Wolff-Parkinson-White syndrome is its tendency to association with attacks of supraventricular tachycardia, particularly of atrial tachycardia but also of atrial fibrillation or flutter. There is probably an even greater tendency to attacks of tachycardia in individuals with a short P-R interval and normal QRS complex,[1] a condition designated by some as "coronary nodal rhythm."[2] This is not to be confused with the "coronary sinus rhythm" of Scherf[3] in which the P waves are inverted in Leads II and III, the P-R interval is not shortened and there is no propensity to paroxysmal tachycardia.

DIAGNOSIS

Occasionally the physician must make the diagnosis from the history. The patient has already recovered from his attack and the physician must do his best to define the disturbance in rhythm on the basis of the patient's description of the attack. He will have to pay particular attention to the heart rate, to the patient's impression of whether the rhythm was regular or irregular, to the manner of onset and offset and to the factor, if any, that seemed responsible for the termination of the attack. Even though the situation is then not truly an emergency, this attempt is well worthwhile for it may permit a presumptive diagnosis. Knowing what sort of an attack a patient has just had may give a reliable clue to what sort of an attack he is likely again to have. At best, however, such a definition is tentative and not so reliable as that made during an attack actually observed.

More commonly the patient is seen in the midst of an attack. The physician has been unable to observe its beginning. The heart rate is rapid, generally varying from 140 to 240, and the rhythm is perfectly regular. (Fig. 15.) Most physicians disclaim ability to count the heart rate at these rapid rates. Actually this is a skill which can quite readily be acquired. One trick which can be recommended is to think or tap in rhythm with the heart, using the mind as a mental Veeder counter. The use of polysyllabic numbers such as eleven (e-le-ven) or twenty (twen-ty) must be eliminated else one loses count. It is convenient to count in ones, accenting the count at multiples of ten as follows:

one-two-three-four-five-six-se-eight, nine, tén,
one-two-three-four-five-six-se-eight-nine-twén

and continuing, using thir for thirty, four for forty, fif for fifty, six for sixty, se for seventy, eight for eighty, nine for ninety and hun for one hundred. In this way a very high degree of accuracy may be attained, allowing an error of two (over the course of a full minute), one for a missed first beat and one for a missed last beat. In paroxysmal atrial tachycardia the rate shows no more than this two point variation when counted repeatedly after minutes even when the patient changes his position or exercises or does something else that would ordinarily be expected to alter his heart rate. Furthermore the heart sounds have precisely the same intensity and quality from cycle to cycle over long periods of observation. Most important of all, and here diagnosis and treatment may be served equally well, stimulation of the carotid sinus either has no effect whatever on the tachycardia or it suddenly terminates the paroxysm. From

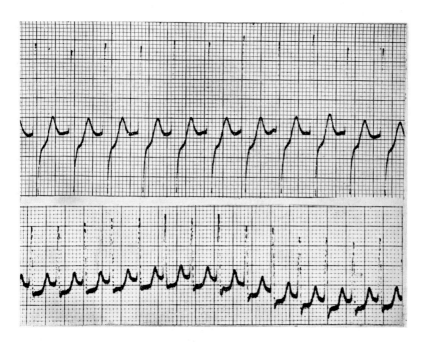

Fig. 15. *Two Cases of Paroxysmal Atrial Tachycardia.* The rhythm is precisely regular in each, the rate 166 in the upper, 214 in the lower tracing. P waves are not identified with certainty. In the upper strip there is pronounced, in the lower moderate, depression of the RS-T segment, attributable to subendocardial ischemia.

a rate of, say, 190, after a short pause, punctuated perhaps by one or more nodal or ventricular premature or escape beats, a normal mechanism returns at a rate of 90 or 100.

There are three rather rare exceptions to the rule that the rhythm is precisely regular in paroxysmal atrial tachycardia. The first is in the short repetitive bouts of atrial tachycardia described by Parkinson and Papp.[4] (Fig. 16.) The second consists of a variety of paroxysmal atrial tachycardia in which there is an alternation in cycle length.[5] (Fig. 17.) And the third is the rare detection of ventricular premature beats in the midst of a paroxysm. In one such attack the extrasystoles were quite frequent. (Fig. 18.) This attack was terminated by ocular pressure.

In the electrocardiogram the P wave is generally a miserable affair. The P-R interval is apt to be prolonged to the upper limits of normal or beyond. Hence the P wave is frequently engulfed in the T wave of the preceding complex. Generally, therefore, a P wave cannot be seen at all. (Fig. 15.) Where transitions are seen in one lead between normal sinus rhythm and paroxysmal atrial tachycardia, it is quite clear that the configuration of the P wave of the paroxysm is different from the normal P wave. (Fig. 16.) Careful caliper examination shows the cycle length to be fixed. Obvious alternation in cycle length has been quite exceptional in my experience. The appearance of the ventricular complex is ordinarily identical with that seen during normal sinus rhythm. But if intraventricular block is already present during normal rhythm this will persist during the paroxysm and thus, to a greater or lesser extent, cause the latter to simulate paroxysmal ventricular tachycardia. Occasionally intraventricular block may be a function of heart rate, bizarre ventricular complexes being recorded only above a certain critical ventricular rate. Here differentiation from ventricular tachycardia may be even more difficult for a normal ventricular complex will be re-

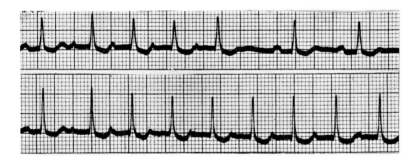

Fig. 16. *"Repetitive" Paroxysmal Atrial Tachycardia* (Parkinson-Papp). The upper strip shows the end of one bout in which the cycle length is inconstant. Lower strip, from same patient, shows another salvo in its entirety. Here the rhythm is regular. In each the P-R interval is slightly lengthened.

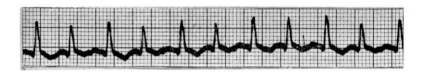

Fig. 17. *Paroxysmal Atrial Tachycardia with Alternation in Cycle Length.*
Noticeable alternation is quite unusual in paroxysmal atrial tachycardia.

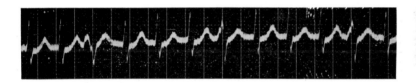

Fig. 18. Ventricular premature beats during paroxysmal atrial tachycardia.

recorded with a slowed ventricular rate and normal sinus rhythm. RS-T segment shifts and T wave changes may develop during the more rapid rhythms. These may be secondary to the rapid rate itself but frequently a characteristic depression of the RS-T segment is recorded with a persistently upright T wave suggesting subendocardial ischemia. (Fig. 15.) That this is not the effect of the rapid rate itself is demonstrated by its occasional persistence over minutes, days, or even weeks after the cessation of a paroxysm.

DIFFERENTIAL DIAGNOSIS

Paroxysmal atrial tachycardia must be distinguished from normal sinus tachycardia, from atrial flutter, from atrial tachycardia with block and from ventricular tachycardia. In sinus tachycardia the heart rate generally varies from 100 to 140 but it may reach 180. A rate between 100 and 140 is more in line with sinus tachycardia, over 140 with paroxysmal atrial tachycardia. The rate is generally not as fixed in sinus tachycardia as in paroxysmal atrial tachycardia. In sinus tachycardia, if the rate is counted repeatedly over the course of five, ten or more minutes (in the manner described above), it may be found to vary by more than 4 beats per minute. Similar observation in atrial tachycardia shows no more variation than 2 per minute. Exercise or change of position produces no change in the heart rate in paroxysmal atrial tachycardia but may induce significant changes in the rate in sinus tachycardia. But there are some cases of sinus tachycardia in which the rate is quite fixed. The onset and offset of sinus tachycardia are gradual; that of paroxysmal auricular tachycardia abrupt. The gradual acceleration and deceleration of the heart in sinus tachycardia may be observed over minutes, hours or days, or in a single electrocardiographic strip.

In sinus tachycardia the P wave of the electrocardiogram has a normal or even an increased amplitude. This results from the migration of the site of impulse formation to a more cephalic position in the sinus node. In sinus tachycardia the P-R interval may increase, but rarely to the degree attained in paroxysmal atrial tachycardia. In many cases there is even a shortening of the P-R interval in sinus tachycardia. This combination of shortened P-R and prominent P wave produces a striking contrast with the minuscule P wave and lengthened P-R of paroxysmal atrial tachycardia. Finally the effect of vagal maneuvers such as stimulation of the carotid sinus is quite different in these two forms of tachycardia. In sinus tachycardia carotid sinus stimulation either has no effect upon the mechanism at all or it induces, over the course of a few beats, slight but smooth and gradual slowing of the heart rate with gradual return to the original rate when the pressure is released. In paroxysmal atrial tachycardia, on the other hand, carotid sinus stimulation either has no effect at all or it induces a prompt and abrupt restoration of normal sinus rhythm. On release of carotid pressure the heart remains in normal rhythm. Thus if this maneuver has no effect upon the heart rate, one cannot be certain of the rhythm; if smooth transient slowing is induced you are dealing with sinus tachycardia, and if the procedure stops the paroxysm, two things have been accomplished; the attack has been both diagnosed and treated as paroxysmal atrial tachycardia.

Atrial flutter In paroxysmal atrial tachycardia the first sound does not change in intensity; in flutter its intensity may or may not vary. In paroxysmal atrial tachycardia the rhythm is perfectly regular; in flutter it may be perfectly regular or "regularly" irregular. A regular rhythm with a rate between 140 and 190 could be either paroxysmal atrial tachycardia or atrial flutter; a rate exceeding 190 is more likely to indicate paroxysmal atrial tachycardia. Carotid sinus stimulation may have no effect upon the ventricular rate in paroxysmal atrial tachycardia or in atrial flutter; if, on the other hand, this procedure terminates the attack, paroxysmal atrial tachycardia was its mechanism. In flutter the rate is only temporarily slowed. On cessation of carotid sinus stimulation the original rate is resumed in the course of a few beats. And finally a classical "saw-tooth" contour is seen in the electrocardiogram in flutter at a glance or with some effort and experience. In paroxysmal atrial tachycardia one sees regular puny P waves or no P waves at all.

Atrial tachycardia with block Partial (second degree) or, much more rarely, complete (third degree) atrioventricular block develops spontaneously or is induced deliberately in atrial tachycardia with block. Until such block develops and while 1:1 conduction is present, one cannot be certain which of the two mechanisms, classical paroxysmal atrial tachycardia or atrial tachycardia with latent block, is present. Atrioventricular block does not develop in garden-variety paroxysmal atrial tachycardia. These two rhythms are further differentiated on the basis of the regularity of the auricular rhythm and of the clinical settings in which they develop. Their differentiation is discussed more fully in the succeeding chapters.

Paroxysmal ventricular tachycardia In atrial tachycardia the rhythm is perfectly regular. In tachycardia of the ventricles the rhythm may be regular or very slightly irregular. This is an irregularity which is detected only on careful auscultation. A regular rhythm may occur therefore in either atrial or ventricular tachycardia. In atrial tachycardia there is no variation in the intensity of the first sound. In most cases of ventricular tachycardia, by contrast, there are such changes. This is the result of the atrioventricular dissociation which is a feature of most cases of ventricular tachycardia and the resultant changes in the time relationships between atrial and ventricular contraction. Where the ventricles are driving the atria (retrograde atrial activation), this phenomenon is not observed and the first sounds do not vary in intensity. Carotid sinus stimulation never stops ventricular tachycardia; it may abolish tachycardia of the auricles. This latter procedure is the only one on the basis of which a definitive clinical differentiation can be made.

In paroxysmal atrial tachycardia P waves may be seen "in the clear" or as a deformity in the T waves of preceding complexes. Each P wave is followed by a ventricular complex. In ventricular tachycardia P waves are difficult to identify. They are apt to produce a deformity of the ventricular complex. Because of changing relationships between auricular and ventricular activation these P waves are inscribed at different moments in the ventricular complex of successive cycles. Frequently they are not identifiable at all. In rare cases of ventricular tachycardia the P waves are closely linked with ventricular complexes. This is particularly true when there is retrograde ventriculo-atrial activation. In uncomplicated atrial tachycardia the QRS complex has a normal duration and is identical with, or very close in appearance to, that of the complexes recorded in the same lead during normal sinus rhythm. In ventricular tachycardia, on the other hand, the ventricular complexes are bizarre, last 0.12 second or longer and, because of superimposition of P waves, generally show a somewhat variable contour from complex to complex. The problem of differentiating between paroxysmal atrial tachycardia and paroxysmal ventricular tachycardia is somewhat more difficult when paroxysmal atrial tachycardia is complicated by intraventricular block. This may be relatively easy to establish if intraventricular block was present before the attack or is demonstrated during normal rhythm after the subsidence of the attack. But in some cases intraventricular block may develop *pari-passu* with the tachycardia. When a P wave can be demonstrated invariably to precede each bizarre ventricular complex one may be very suspicious that one is dealing with supraventricular tachycardia complicated by intraventricular block. In some cases stimulation of the carotid sinus, by aborting the attack, makes it clear that the mechanism was paroxysmal atrial tachycardia. In others no change is produced. One may then still remain in doubt. In still others carotid sinus stimulation slows the atria, not the ventricles. This then is clearly paroxysmal ventricular tachycardia. In many, definite differentiation between the two is not possible.

TREATMENT

The long-run prophylaxis of paroxysmal atrial tachycardia is not an emergency consideration and does not concern us here. Neither need an acute paroxysm necessarily constitute an emergency. Many attacks can be treated by simply having the patient lie down and possibly take a sedative. Very often the patient will have learned some "little trick" whereby he can stop his own attack. Among the various "vagal" maneuvers which may stop an attack are the taking and holding of a deep breath, compression of the abdomen, bending over in certain positions, bearing down against a closed glottis (Valsalva maneuver) as in the act of defecation, drinking ice water or swallowing ice. To be effective it is apparently necessary that the stimulation, in the words of Soma Weiss, be "deep."

If these simple personal measures have been unsuccessful the physician himself should try to stop the attack with carotid sinus stimulation. One should feel for the bulge at the bifurcation of the common carotid artery just below the angle of the jaw and, with a rotary motion, press this structure against the cervical spine for a period of about five seconds. Often this will abruptly revert an attack to normal rhythm. If this is ineffective one should try a corresponding region on the other side of the neck. If this in turn is ineffective one should return to the original side and try a little higher. Then a little higher on the opposite side. Then, if still without effect, a little lower on one side, then on the other. In this way numerous areas will have been tried on each side persistently. The two sides should never be stimulated simultaneously. Particularly in elderly patients such practice, presumably by effectively throttling cerebral blood flow, has led to cerebral thrombosis. For the same reason stimulation should not be continued for longer than five seconds at a time. This is true whether this procedure is employed for diagnostic or therapeutic purposes. Carotid sinus stimulation rarely aborts attacks in children.[6]

If carotid sinus stimulation is ineffective, one may try ocular pressure ("oculo-cardiac reflex"). If the patient is conscious, this will be painful but the procedure has been successful in fully anaesthetized patients. Pressure is applied, again over a period of five seconds or so, first to one eyeball, then, if ineffective, to the other. In extremely rare instances this procedure has produced detachment of the retina. In view of this reported experience, it would probably be wise to avoid this procedure in myopic individuals.[7] Sometimes "pulling the tongue out by its roots" is effective. This is done in the manner of the laryngoscopic examination, wrapping the tongue with a gauze strip, handkerchief or towel and pulling firmly outwards. Occasionally gagging the patient by tickling the back of his throat with a tongue depressor or finger, even to the point of making him vomit, will stop an attack. Or he can be made to vomit by having him drink a little mustard water or a teaspoonful or two of tincture of ipecac. Some writers have suggested the subcutaneous injection of 5 mgms. of apomorphine but I have never had the heart to use it.

If these simple "vagal" maneuvers have been ineffective and it seems from the condition of the patient that the attack should not be allowed to continue, one may use various medicinal forms of treatment. Probably the simplest and most effective is the subcutaneous injection of 0.5 to 1.0 or even

2.0 mgms. of Prostigmine. Two possible side-effects of this medication are the development of abdominal cramps or diarrhoea and the precipitation of an asthmatic attack. Therefore this drug should be avoided in the presence of abdominal obstruction or in the face of a history of bronchial asthma or allergic diseases.

Another choice of medication is digitalis. In a previously undigitalized patient this may be given intravenously in the form of Digoxin (1.0 mgm.) or Cedilanid (0.8-1.2 mgm.). In patients who have already received some digitalis smaller doses (0.5 mgm. Digoxin or 0.4 mgm. Cedilanid) may be used as an initial dose. If the attack is not thus aborted, increments of 0.25 mgm. of Digoxin or 0.4 mgm. of Cedilanid may be given at two-hourly intervals. Nadas [8] recommends that a child less than two years old be given, as an initial parenteral dose 0.02 to 0.03 mgm. of either Digoxin or Cedilanid per pound of body weight, or 0.01 to 0.02 mgm. per pound to a child two years of age or older. Because of the possibility of future recurrences it should be borne in mind that any treatment of paroxysmal atrial tachycardia is a titration for future reference. Therefore the use of a rapidly acting intravenous digitalis preparation is preferred. Its effect is total and convincing. On the other hand, if quinidine is given by mouth in repetitive doses, as is commonly practiced, it may be very difficult to be sure whether reversion has been induced by quinidine or has occurred spontaneously. Although quinidine by mouth has been commonly recommended for paroxysmal atrial tachycardia, there is, then, this practical objection to its employment. Quinidine or Pronestyl may be given by mouth (page 227) if digitalis is ineffective, or by vein (page 279) if the condition of the patient has become desperate.

Mecholyl chloride (Acetyl-beta-methyl choline chloride) 20 mgm. injected subcutaneously is very commonly recommended for paroxysmal atrial tachycardia. But this injection is so frequently followed by a seemingly endless period of asystole before the normal pacemaker reasserts its control of the heart mechanism, that I have preferred not to use it. Its use is proscribed in allergic or asthmatic individuals. Atropine should always be at hand when it is used. Mention has just been made of the standstill which may follow Mecholyl therapy. A short period of asystole is, in fact, a regular feature of the termination of most attacks of atrial tachycardia. And a rare individual has been known to have his tachycardia stopped but not followed by resumption of a heart beat, simply because of failure of re-emergence of a normal pacemaker. In this situation a brisk blow to the precordium with the fist or the heel of the hand may start the heart beating again. If this is ineffective the use, if available, of a cardiac "pacemaker" or thoracotomy with manual systole and the employment of procedures aiming at the resuscitation of cardiac pacemakers, may be imperative. (page 338).

If the patient has developed a moderate to profound drop in blood pressure pressor amines should be given as in shock. Corday [9] prefers to begin this form of treatment immediately after the mechanical measures described above have been found to be ineffective, maintaining the blood pressure at a normal level until other antiarrhythmic drugs have taken effect. His preference is to nor-epinephrine by intravenous drip. Over and above this effect of the pressor amines in making possible a more leisurely treatment of atrial tachycardia, there is evidence that these drugs, of themselves, possess some antiarrhythmic properties. Mephentermine,[10] neo-synephrine and Vasoxyl,[11] presumably in part at least by virtue of their effect in increasing the pressure in the aortic arch and its branches and thereby in stimulating the aortic baroreceptors, has stopped attacks in one or two minutes and may be worthy of trial. The medical literature also reports the successful use of calcium gluconate (10 to 20 cc. of a 10% solution given slowly by vein). Quinacrine hydrochloride (Atabrine) enjoyed a brief vogue in the treatment of paroxysmal tachycardia after World War II. The dose is 0.1 gram of 1% solution by vein or 0.3 gram in 1% procaine solution intramuscularly.[12]

It is well to remember, if any of these various medications has not in itself abolished the arrhythmia, that super-added carotid sinus stimulation applied at the time of expected maximum physiological effect of the drug (generally 20 to 30 minutes after its administration) may be followed by reversion.

Where a definite decision between paroxysmal ventricular tachycardia and paroxysmal atrial tachycardia with intraventricular block has not been possible, quinidine or Pronestyl may be tried as a first tack. Since magnesium is apparently equally effective against atrial and ventricular tachycardia, magnesium sulfate, 4 cc. of a 50% solution or 20 cc. of a 20% solution may be injected intravenously under these same circumstances.

For the chest pain that may accompany paroxysmal tachycardia the important indication, of course, is to terminate the attack. But I have seen occasional cases in which I could not immediately stop the attack but in which the chest pain was alleviated or eliminated by nitroglycerin while the paroxysm continued.

Paroxysmal nodal tachycardia The inherent rate of the atrioventricular node varies from 35 to 60. Thus when the atrioventricular node drives the heart the rate does not exceed the latter figure. This is true nodal rhythm. A rate between 60 and 100 might be considered *nodal tachycardia*. This is not *paroxysmal* nodal tachycardia. But where the site of impulse formation is in the node and the rate exceeds 100 or attains that seen in paroxysmal atrial tachycardia, one is dealing with *paroxysmal nodal tachycardia*. This condition behaves in all respects like paroxysmal atrial tachycardia but shows inverted P waves in Leads II, III and aVF. In an established attack it

[208]

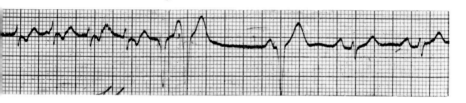

Fig. 19. *Paroxysmal Nodal Tachycardia* stopped with right carotid sinus stimulation. The last QRS of the attack is followed by an inverted (retrograde) P
wave. This is followed by two ventricular premature beats, then, after a pause,
by a non-conducted but upright P wave and then a ventricular escape beat.
Then follows resumption of normal sinus rhythm. If the last QRS of the
paroxysm were not followed by an inverted P wave this would be paroxysmal
atrial tachycardia.

is impossible to say whether this inverted P wave is conducted in a retrograde direction from the preceding QRS complex or is conducted to the succeeding QRS complex. It has been considered that one can settle this issue by observing the beginning or end of a paroxysm. If the bout starts with a P wave preceding the QRS complex and shows no retrograde P wave at the end of an attack, one is dealing with paroxysmal atrial tachycardia. If the bout starts with a QRS complex and ends with a retrograde P wave, (Fig. 19) paroxysmal nodal tachycardia should be diagnosed. I have seen an occasional attack in which an upright P wave initiates and an inverted P wave terminates the paroxysm. This raises some interesting theoretical points which are not germane to this discussion. One can only say that as a practical consideration it does not matter whether the mechanism is paroxysmal atrial tachycardia or paroxysmal nodal tachycardia. The treatment is the same in either case.

REFERENCES

(1) Lown, B., Ganong, W. F. and Levine, S. A.: The syndrome of short P-R interval, normal QRS complex and paroxysmal rapid heart action. Circ. 5: 693, 1952.

(2) Katz, L. N. and Pick, A.: Clinical Electrocardiography. Part I. The Arrhythmias. Lea and Febiger, Philadelphia, 1956, p. 102.

(3) Scherf, D. and Harris, R.: Coronary sinus rhythm. Am. Ht. J. 32: 443, 1946.

(4) Parkinson, J. and Papp, C.: Repetitive paroxysmal tachycardia. Brit. Ht. J. 9: 21, 1947.

(5) Barker, P. S., Johnston, F. D. and Wilson, F. N.: Auricular paroxysmal tachycardia with alternation of cycle length. Am. Ht. J. 25: 799, 1943.

(6) Langendorf, R. and Pick, A.: Cardiac arrhythmias in infants and children. Ped. Clin. No. Am. Feb. 1954, p. 215.

(7) Scherf, D.: Clinical progress. Treatment of cardiac arrhythmias. Circulation 8: 756, 1953.

(8) Nadas, A. S.: Pediatric Cardiology. W. B. Saunders
Company. Philadelphia and London, 1957, p. 184.

(9) Corday, E., Gold H., de Vrea, L. B., Williams, J. H. and
Fields, J.: Effect of the cardiac arrhythmias on the coronary circulation. Ann. Int. Med. 50: 535, 1959.

(10) Bernstein, A., Cohen, F., Robins, B. and Simon, F.: The
treatment of arrhythmias and shock with mephentermine
in large doses. J. Newark Beth Israel Hospital. 9: 3, 1958.

(11) Nathanson, M. H. and Miller, H.: Clinical observations
on a new epinephrine-like compound, Methoxamine, Am.
J. Med. Sci. 223: 270, 1952.

(12) Gertler, M. M. and Yohalem, S. B.: Effect of quinacrine
on auricular fibrillation and tachycardia. J. Mt. Sinai
Hosp. 10: 297, 1947.

10

ATRIAL FLUTTER

Differential Diagnosis

Treatment

10

ATRIAL FLUTTER

When the ventricular rate is neither rapid nor unduly slow, atrial flutter or fibrillation is not serious. On the contrary, with a rapid ventricular rate either of these arrhythmias may constitute an acute emergency. The treatment of choice for atrial flutter under these circumstances is to slow the heart with digitalis. Therapy is therefore generally simple and straightforward. Diagnosis, by contrast, is often quite difficult. Although there are many reliable bedside clues to its presence, the diagnosis of flutter is made, in the last analysis, by the electrocardiogram. An understanding of the electrocardiographic features of this disturbance moreover anticipates and explains its many clinical vagaries. Therefore, an exposition of the electrocardiographic features of flutter is presented at the outset.

The electrocardiographic diagnosis depends principally upon the detection of a characteristic continuous undulation of the baseline between ventricular complexes. This generally shows a fairly abrupt upstroke and a more gradual and hesitant downstroke. (Fig. 20.) The resultant configuration has been likened to a saw-tooth but at times the appearance may be sinusoidal, triangular or scalloped, (Fig. 20,E) and lack the characteristic pause on the downstroke. At other times the horizontal segment may be quite long and, in series, produce an appearance resembling a succession of plateaus flanked by sharp peaks. These

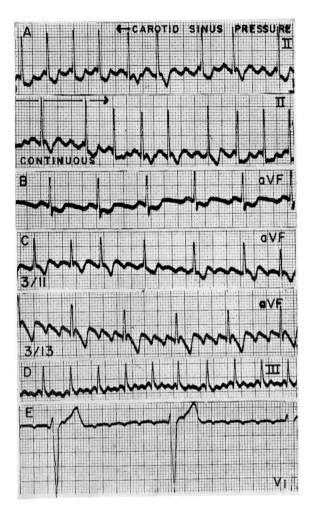

Fig. 20. *Contour of Baseline and Various Degrees of Atrioventricular Block in Atrial Flutter.* (A) Effect of carotid sinus stimulation on flutter with 2:1 response. Period of stimulation indicated by arrow. The ventricles are slowed revealing continuous flutter contour of baseline. Note "jerky" return to original rate following release of pressure. (B) Classical flutter contour at slow flutter rate (170). 2:1 response. (C) Upper strip shows atrial flutter with variable ventricular response. Note that the cycle length from first to second and from sixth to seventh ventricular beats is equal and that the interval from the third to the sixth ventricular beats is just four times that interval. Thus there is an underlying regularity of the auricles. Lower strip recorded two days later in same patient shows 4:1 response. (D) Atrial flutter with 2:1 response. There is a fine precise undulation whose descending limb shows a slightly rising rather than a level interruption. (E) Atrial flutter with complete heart block. Note scalloped contour of baseline.

[216]

undulations are generally best seen in Leads II, III and aVF, rarely only in Lead V $_1$. In this lead the continuous oscillations of the baseline are generally poorly seen. Instead one sees a prominent rapid deflection ("intrinsicoid deflection"), the result of the closer approximation of the electrode to the auricles. (Fig. 21,A.) Occasionally classical flutter waves are not seen in the extremity leads at all but flutter is demonstrated by regular deflections of this type in Lead V_1 or V_1 and V_2.

Flutter activity is perfectly regular and averages about 300 times per minute (range generally 250 to 350). Because of the physiological inability of the conduction tissues to respond to every impulse at this rapid atrial rate, the ventricles, in the untreated individual, respond to every other beat (2:1 response or 2:1 block). (Fig. 20,A,D.) If the atria are being activated 300 times per minute the resulting ventricular rate would be 150. Higher degrees of block may occur spontaneously or as the result of digitalis therapy. If there is a 4:1 response the ventricular rate would be 75, if a variable response, the ventricular rhythm would be irregular. Although this is often referred to loosely as a "grossly irregular" rhythm this description is inaccurate. Because the underlying atrial mechanism remains perfectly regular throughout, there is a fundamental persistent background regularity to the ventricular rhythm. Although some of the ventricular deflections may be a little "off the beat," too many of them occur just on time to be attributable to chance. ("Regular irregularity.") (Fig. 20,C.) This is not observed in atrial fibrillation.

With the more rapid ventricular rates seen in the emergency situations under discussion the classical flutter contour may be obscured by the ventricular complexes and it may be difficult to distinguish a free flutter wave, or part of a free flutter wave, from a P, R or T wave. With experience it is possible mentally to "extrapolate" continuous auricular activity through the ven-

[217]

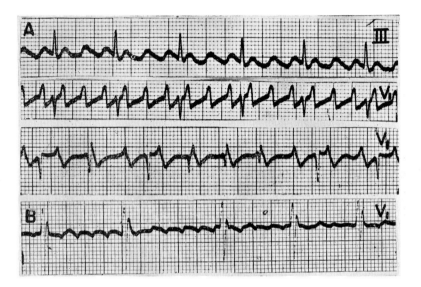

Fig. 21. *Atrial Flutter.* (A) Difference in baseline contour between extremity and chest leads. Flutter with 3:1 response. Flutter rate 275. Note classical contour in Lead III. In Lead V_1 large "intrinsicoid deflections" are superimposed upon a triangular baseline. Two days later the flutter rate has slowed to 176. At this time there is a periodic 1:1 response in the middle of the strip. (B) Impure flutter. Caliper examination shows that the "flutter" rate is not perfectly regular. The uniform appearance of the first half of the strip is lost in the second half.

[218]

tricular complexes. This technique of suspicion is particularly applicable in 2:1 block. Here it is often helpful to draw in the hidden second undulation which coincides in part with the QRS complex. In rare cases ventricular activity may be isoelectric or nearly isoelectric in one lead, e.g. Lead III or aVF. In this instance pure auricular activity—and nothing but flutter waves—may be seen in this lead. When there is doubt about the nature of auricular activity the carotid sinus should be stimulated for a few seconds during a recording of Lead II, III, aVF or V 1, whichever looks more promising. The technique of this procedure is described on page 204. Where this is successful the degree of block is increased, fewer flutter waves are followed by ventricular complexes and the characteristic undulant contour of flutter may be clearly displayed during the lengthened intervals thus produced between ventricular complexes. Carotid sinus stimulation is helpful in the diagnosis of flutter in another way. Its effect upon the ventricular rate is only temporary. During, and for a short period after this procedure, the ventricular rate is slowed. On release of carotid pressure the original ventricular rate is resumed in the course of several beats. Characteristically the restitution of the original rate is a "jerky" affair with some longer and shorter intervals being interspersed. (Fig. 20,A.) Rarely the return to the rapid ventricular rate is a "smooth" process with progressive shortening of the ventricular cycle.

At times, particularly in children and in patients receiving quinidine (which has the effect of enhancing atrioventricular conduction), the ventricles may respond to every atrial impulse. This is the so-called 1:1 response. This state is generally poorly tolerated for, if persistent, this rate may precipitate congestive heart failure or collapse. This is one reason why it is good practice thoroughly to digitalize patients with flutter before proceeding with quinidine therapy. By producing a greater degree of block at the atrioventricular level the effect of quinidine in enhancing atrioventricular conduction is antagonized. (Fig. 22.)

While electrocardiographic confirmation is always desirable, the presence of atrial flutter may be first suspected or established on the basis of certain bedside observations.[1] At times an electrocardiographic machine may not be available or usable. When the existence of flutter has already been documented, the continued presence of this arrhythmia may likewise be demonstrated by similar clinical methods without the need for more than a few electrocardiograms. Some of these clues have already been described in the discussion of the electrocardiogram and may frequently be as readily appreciated by careful auscultation as by graphic means. Among them are the transient response of the ventricles to carotid sinus stimulation, the "jerky" return and the dominant underlying regularity of the cardiac rhythm when the ventricles are irregular. A physician with a well developed sense of rhythm can often detect this regularity almost instinctively. Others can learn to appreciate this pattern by the simple device of tapping the foot or a pencil in rhythm with the heart and noting the frequent coincidence of the heart beat with these tappings.

Variations in sympathetic-parasympathetic tone can produce changes in the responsiveness of the atrioventricular conduction tissue. When the responsiveness is thus enhanced, as for example by exercise, a critical level of conductibility may be exceeded. If the original rate is 75 and the rhythm regular, there may then be an abrupt doubling of the heart rate to 150. This would be the result of a change from 4:1 to 2:1 response. It is, of course, this very phenomenon which explains the extreme and frequently disabling lability of the heart rate in atrial flutter. And in some patients, particularly those with heart disease, this change may be tantamount to the development or exacerbation of dyspnea, congestive failure, chest pain or syncope. Sometimes exercising the patient enables one

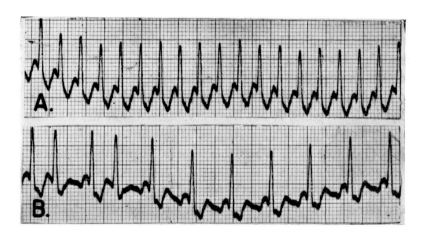

Fig. 22. *Atrial Flutter with 1:1 Response.* (Ld. II) Attempt had first been made to revert patient to normal mechanism with quinidine alone. On development of 1:1 response patient went into collapse. Lower strip shows spontaneous change to 2:1 response when patient felt better. On discontinuing quinidine, then digitalizing patient, subsequent quinidinization induced uneventful reversion to sinus rhythm.

to distinguish the "irregular" ventricular rhythm of flutter from that of fibrillation. In atrial fibrillation, if the ventricular rate is, say, 72 and the rhythm irregular, exercise might accelerate the ventricles but their rhythm would remain grossly irregular. In atrial flutter, on the other hand, exercise would be expected to make the ventricles rapid, say, 150, and perfectly regular. Generally these patients can tolerate the mild degree of exercise, for example a few trunk bends, necessary to demonstrate this response.

Physical examination may disclose two other findings which are helpful in making the diagnosis. The first of these is the detection on auscultation at the cardiac apex of striking changes in the intensity of the first heart sound when the ventricular rhythm is irregular. It has been emphasized that the intensity of the first sound is a function of atrioventricular conduction time (P-R interval). When this interval is prolonged beyond 0.20 second the first sound is generally decreased in intensity or may even be absent. When the interval ranges between 0.15 and 0.19 second, it is generally normal in intensity; when shortened below 0.15 second, the first sound is accentuated and at times may be booming in quality. The pronounced variability in the intensity of S_1 in atrial flutter with an irregular rhythm is due to the changing interval from flutter wave to ventricular contraction with successive cycles. There may be some variability in S_1 in many cases of atrial fibrillation but this is not so striking as that heard in flutter. The second clue from physical examination is the presence of flutter waves in the neck veins. Since the atrial rhythm remains perfectly regular and undisturbed no matter what the ventricles do, one may observe regular pulsations in the jugular veins at a rate of, say, 300. Careful inspection of the neck may show two venous pulsations for each arterial wave. This might consist of two distinct fillings of the neck veins for each single lift of the neck structures imparted by the deeper and more forceful carotid pulsation, or of two distinct venous pulsations for each heart beat heard over the precordium. In this case there must be a 2:1 response. Alternatively one might see regular flutter waves in the neck while the ventricles beat irregularly; this corresponds to atrial flutter with variable ventricular response.

The detection of these phenomena from physical examination requires considerable practice and assiduous application on the part of the observer. With the ubiquitous electrocardiograph, the present-day tendency to the machine-made diagnosis, and the lazy excuse that the tracing serves, in any event, as a permanent record of the arrhythmia, this is an aspect of cardiac diagnosis which is generally neglected. This is unfortunate for, particularly where serial observations are necessary, a decision regarding the arrhythmia may frequently be made with the aid of these bedside maneuvers without involving the patient in the expense of innumerable electrocardiograms.

DIFFERENTIAL DIAGNOSIS

Atrial flutter must be differentiated from atrial fibrillation, from classical paroxysmal atrial tachycardia, from atrial tachycardia with block and from paroxysmal ventricular tachycardia. Flutter is distinguished from fibrillation of the auricles by the characteristic contour of the baseline and the precise regularity of the auricular rhythm. Fibrillation by contrast shows a varying contour with smaller atrial deflections ("f" waves) and variable intervals between individual fibrillation waves. The latter are much shorter than flutter waves, their rate varying from 350 to 500 or greater. In fibrillation the ventricular rhythm is grossly ("irregularly") irregular. In flutter the ventricular rhythm may be regular or irregular. When irregular there is a background of dominant regularity ("regularly irregular"). Differentiation between these two mechanisms on the basis of their response to exercise and to carotid sinus stimulation and of the different degree of changes in the intensity of the first sound has already been mentioned. At times the contour of the baseline may be quite classical for flutter but the auricular rhythm is very slightly irregular. One may then be dealing with a mechanism intermediate between atrial flutter and fibrillation. This may be termed "impure flutter," (Fig. 21,B), "flutter-fibrillation," "fibrillo-flutter" or "coarse fibrillation," depending upon one's semantics. At times the atrial mechanism may shade from a perfectly regular atrial rhythm to an irregular atrial disturbance with very similar morphology. At other times the atria may kaleidoscope from one mechanism to another. Thus during the recording of the usual twelve leads one may record flutter in some leads, fibrillation in others and even normal sinus rhythm in still others. One may even see transitions from one rhythm to another in a single lead. This tendency to metamorphosis often confuses the picture but there is no serious practical problem in the differentiation of these two rhythms for the treatment of one is the treatment of the other.

The differentiation between atrial flutter and paroxysmal atrial tachycardia is discussed in the preceding chapter (page 201). At times a differentiation cannot be made even with the aid of the electrocardiograph. Here the non-commital designation "supraventricular tachycardia, type undetermined" may be all that is justified.

In the presence of intraventricular block atrial flutter with a rapid ventricular rate may be confused with ventricular tachycardia. The problem is simplified if previous or subsequent tracings recorded during normal sinus rhythm show intraventricular block and ventricular complexes identical with or very similar to those seen during the tachycardia. One would then be justified in assuming that this is a supraventricular tachycardia with the same persistent type of intraventricular block. Even when the ventricular rate is rapid it is often possible to detect or suspect the characteristic flutter contour in the background. Occasionally intraventricular block is a factor of the heart rate. When a certain critical ventricular rate is exceeded the ventricular complexes may resemble right or left bundle branch block. Below that rate the ventricular complexes show a normal QRS duration. Under these circumstances carotid sinus stimulation, by slowing the ventricular response, may not only reveal flutter waves but may also disclose "normal" ventricular complexes at the slowed rate. Such slowing does not occur in ventricular tachycardia. If carotid pressure is without effect one may have to remain in doubt. Since flutter with 1:1 response is frequently associated with intraventricular block, and since carotid sinus stimulation is often ineffective in 1:1 flutter, the differentiation from ventricular tachycardia may be difficult or impossible.

The differentiation between atrial flutter and atrial tachycardia with block is one of the most difficult of arrhythmia problems. This is discussed at length in the succeeding chapter (page 238).

These ideas are at some variance with present thinking regarding the unity of all atrial arrhythmias. It has been shown [2,3] for example that chemical or electrical stimulation of the heart of the experimental animal seems to be capable of inducing various atrial disturbances whose form apparently depends upon the rate and site of impulse formation. With rapid rates and a site of origin low in the auricles, the resultant rhythm resembles human atrial flutter. With a slow rate and a point of origin of the impulse high in the atria, the disturbance resembles paroxysmal atrial tachycardia. Atrial tachycardia with block would, by inference, be a mechanism intermediary between these two. The clinical implication is that these are all fundamentally alike, that they differ only in detail, and that the management of one is the management of all. In point of fact, however, the treatment of flutter is diametrically opposite that of most cases of atrial tachycardia with block. Thus, although we may eventually be compelled to surrender the time-honored ideas of their mechanisms, empirical experience justifies their differentiation.

TREATMENT

Atrial flutter with a rapid ventricular rate may be an acute emergency. The immediate concern of the physician is to slow the ventricles by increasing the degree of block with digitalis. Quinidine has no place in the immediate treatment of flutter.[4] Route and dosage of digitalis depend upon the assessed urgency of the situation. Where the condition of the patient is satisfactory slow digitalization by mouth over the course of 24 or 48 hours may be all that is necessary. The fact that fairly rapid digitalization can be achieved orally does not appear to be generally appreciated. One may give digitalis leaf 0.4 to 0.8 gram as an initial dose, then 0.2 gram every four hours for several doses. If significant slowing of the ventricles or anorexia or nausea have not developed by this time, one may "close down" in this process of digitalization by continuing with 0.2 or 0.1 gram t.i.d. until the "end point" of therapeutic or minor toxic effect is attained. Alternatively one may initiate therapy with Digoxin 1.0 mgm. then give 0.5 mgm. as a second or third dose four and eight hours later, completing the procedure similarly with 0.25 to 0.5 mgm. t.i.d. There are many other satisfactory digitalis preparations. These two preparations are listed here merely because I am most familiar with them. When the condition of the patient is desperate, rapid intravenous digitalization may be mandatory. Unfortunately the decision regarding urgency is occasionally determined by the temperament of the physician or the importunity of the patient's family rather than by the condition of the patient. The need for rapid intravenous digitalization is rare in clinical practice. The details of this procedure are given on page 255. Once ventricular slowing has been accomplished, flutter may persist or it may be replaced by atrial fibrillation or even normal sinus rhythm. The management of flutter or fibrillation from this point on does not fall properly within the province of this discussion. Where slowing has not been attained by oral digitalis, and there is any question about absorption, digitalis should be given parenterally.

If the rate still remains rapid resort may have to be had to quinidine therapy in the effort to produce reversion to a normal sinus rhythm. This drug should not be used until it appears likely that the patient is fully digitalized. He should then be kept on maintenance doses of digitalis. The choice between oral and parenteral quinidine therapy will again depend upon the seriousness of the patient's condition. If the drug is to be given by mouth it is given at four-hourly intervals, starting with 0.2 gram and increasing at each dose by 0.1 gram. Thus during the first day of treatment the dosage would be 0.2, 0.3, 0.4, 0.5 and perhaps 0.6 gram. On the following day one may give 0.7, 0.8, 0.9, 1.0, and 1.1 grams as individual doses again at four hourly intervals. If necessary, the dosage, somewhere along here, may be increased by 0.2 rather than 0.1 gram at successive doses. Increasing in either way one may even give up to 2.0 grams in a single dose. It is frequently taught that a single dose of 0.2 gram of the drug should be given by mouth on the eve of the planned treatment. This is intended to detect any idiosyncrasy to the drug. This is generally an unnecessary ritual which, if really done as prescribed, wastes potentially valuable time, particularly in relation to the emergencies here considered. In point of fact, the initial dose in the series 0.2, 0.3, 0.4 gram, etc., should be regarded as the test dose and will as readily reveal the rare instances of idiosyncrasy to the drug as the single "test dose" technique.

At intervals during the process of attempted reversion one determines by clinical and electrocardiographic examination whether reversion to normal sinus rhythm or the development of quinidine toxicity has occurred. Further increments of the drug should not be given if the patient develops ventricular premature beats or abnormal ventricular beats related to the Ashman phenomenon (p. 180), ventricular tachycardia or pronounced hypotension. Some patients receiving moderate to large doses of quinidine complain of an awesome sense of unreality and beg to have the drug discontinued. I suspect that this is really the effect of deafness and a resultant sense of separation from one's surroundings. Deafness, tinnitus and pronounced intraventricular block (QRS prolonged by 50% over the pre-treatment measurement) should be considered relative contraindications to continuing the drug. Where the condition of the patient is desperate, however, cautious increase in dosage may be hazarded in spite of marked widening of the QRS complex and reversion to normal rhythm may yet be attained. During the course of quinidine therapy the flutter rate slows. The auricular rate may fall as low as 150. One effect of this slowing is the "acceptance" by the atrioventricular conduction tissues of a larger proportion of these atrial impulses. At the same time atrioventricular conductibility itself may be enhanced. The combined effect of these two processes may be actually to speed up the ventricles. Such ventricular acceleration during quinidine treatment is apt to alarm the physician and intimidate him against the further use of the drug. Where reversion seems mandatory for the survival of the patient however, this development should not deter him from pushing further increments. Once reversion has been induced no further increases in dosage are given, but one may then institute maintenance quinidine therapy (0.2 to 0.4 gram t.i.d. or q.i.d.) to prevent relapses of flutter.

The use of progressively increasing doses of quinidine as

described above is predicated upon the general premise that physiological effect is correlated roughly with the serum concentration of quinidine. Peak concentration and maximal physiological effect are attained in two hours. Most of a single dose is excreted by four hours but there is some persistence of effect for 24 hours. Used in the manner described above there is undoubtedly some persistence of the effect of a previous dose during the period of the effect of a subsequent dose. The same is true of the alternative technique of giving an identical dose, say 0.4 gram at four-hourly intervals, as is sometimes practiced or, more particularly, at two-hourly intervals.[5] By any of these methods there is a "pyramiding" effect due to accumulation from previous doses.

The measurement of serum quinidine levels by the photofluorometric method has recently been offered [5] as a safer, more useful and more rational guide to the use of the drug, facilitating the determination of optimal dose schedules and helping in the decision whether larger doses of quinidine are justified. With this technique it has been shown that one individual may develop an entirely different serum quinidine level than another on the same dose of the drug. One cannot therefore predict serum level from dosage. It has been my experience, however, that while knowledge of the serum level may provide the clinician with some measure of comfort and security during the process of reversion, as a practical matter this can as safely be accomplished with careful clinical and electrocardiographic observation. Electrocardiographs are now generally available; photofluorometers are not. The information offered by the electrocardiogram is at hand immediately with a direct writing machine; there may be some delay in a serum quinidine level report. It is the effect of the drug at the myocardial cell, not the serum level of the drug, that concerns the physician. The inception of ventricular premature beats would be a danger flag no matter what the serum quinidine level. Thus the lack of

[229]

a photofluorometer need certainly not deter the conscientious clinician from proceeding with the attempt to revert this arrhythmia, or any arrhythmia, with quinidine. Conversion moreover is not necessarily correlated with serum quinidine level. The experience of reversion during the night, hours after the last dose, when the serum level must have been falling, is not uncommon.

On rare occasions it is necessary to administer quinidine parenterally as an emergency measure in atrial flutter. If during the attempted reversion with oral quinidine, the condition of the patient should deteriorate, resort may be had to intravenous or intramuscular therapy with the drug. The details of this treatment are given in the chapter on ventricular tachycardia, page 279.

Where one has been unable to differentiate between atrial flutter and classical paroxysmal atrial tachycardia there is no therapeutic problem. In either case the drug of choice is digitalis. If this is ineffective, quinidine may be tried. The same is true where one is in doubt whether atrial flutter or fibrillation is present. But where doubt exists between atrial flutter on the one hand and atrial tachycardia with block on the other, one is confronted with a difficult clinical situation. While digitalis is preferred for flutter, it is contraindicated in most cases of atrial tachycardia with block, particularly in the type of case being considered here, namely where this disturbance constitutes an acute emergency. This problem is considered in detail in the succeeding chapter (page 238).

Where differentiation has not been possible between atrial flutter with intraventricular block and paroxysmal ventricular tachycardia, quinidine or Pronestyl would likewise be the first choice in therapy. Here one would run the risk of 1:1 response. If the quinidine tack is unsuccessful and the patient is doing badly, one may be justified in doing a complete turnabout to a full-fledged effort at digitalizing the patient. In situations of this type, then, one proceeds on the basis of clinical likelihood, through "trial and error," taking the minimal risk before the maximal risk. If the "safe" drugs are ineffective and the condition of the patient remains or becomes precarious, "risky" procedures or drugs may be justified.

REFERENCES

(1) Levine, S. A.: The bedside recognition and treatment of cardiac irregularities. Internat. Clinics. *4* (Series 46): 161, 1936.
(2) Scherf, D., Roman, F. J. and Terranova, R.: Experimental studies on auricular flutter and auricular fibrillation. Am. Ht. J. *36*: 241, 1948.
(3) Prinzmetal, M. et al. The Auricular Arrhythmias. Charles C. Thomas, Springfield, Illinois, 1952.
(4) Tandowsky, R. M., Oyster, J. M. and Silverglade, A.: The combined use of Lanatoside C and quinidine sulfate in the abolition of established auricular flutter. Am. Ht. J. *32*: 617, 1946.
(5) Sokolow, M. and Ball, R. E.: Factors influencing conversion of chronic atrial fibrillation with special reference to serum quinidine concentration. Circ. *14*: 568, 1956.

11

ATRIAL TACHYCARDIA WITH BLOCK

Electrocardiographic Features

Differential Diagnosis

Management

11

ATRIAL TACHYCARDIA WITH

BLOCK

In about three quarters of cases atrial tachycardia with block is a poorly tolerated arrhythmia. In this group the disorder presents a serious threat to the survival of the patient and demands prompt recognition and appropriate therapy. These patients are already gravely ill with congestive heart failure and possibly shock, acute cor pulmonale or electrolyte imbalance and commonly demonstrate other clinical or electro-cardiographic stigmata of digitalis intoxication.[1] On such a background the inception of atrial tachycardia with block may be hardly, or not at all, noticed. On the other hand, the onset of the arrhythmia may be the very occasion for the first de-velopment of, or for the worsening of, symptoms of congestive heart failure. The deterioration of the patient at this juncture is all too commonly attributed not to the new cardiac mechanism but to pathologic processes known long to be present. In the remaining quarter of cases there need be no heart disease at all, the arrhythmia is quite well tolerated and digitalis is not implicated in its development.

ELECTROCARDIOGRAPHIC FEATURES

This arrhythmia cannot be diagnosed without the electrocardiograph. But this must be subserved by an intelligent appraisal of the clinical background in which it has developed.[2] Atrial tachycardia with block resembles classical paroxysmal atrial tachycardia in some respects, atrial flutter in others. As in the former, the atrial rate generally ranges from about 150 to 200 but may occasionally reach 250 or so. As in the latter arrhythmia, vagal maneuvers fail to abolish the abnormal mechanism but, rather, induce atrioventricular block or increase its degree. In atrial tachycardia with block the electrocardiogram must show an iso-electric baseline between the individual atrial deflections. This is arbitrary and empirical. If a continuously undulating saw-tooth-like baseline is seen, even if only in a single lead, the arrhythmia is atrial flutter, not atrial tachycardia with block.

In atrial tachycardia with block the rhythm of the auricles may be perfectly regular or slightly irregular. In the overwhelming majority of cases the P waves differ from the normal P waves seen previously or subsequently in the same lead. The P waves are generally sharp but may be notched or dome shaped; they may be tall or short but are generally narrow. In some patients the tachycardia may begin and end abruptly and thus be truly paroxysmal. But in most observed attacks, particularly those due to digitalis, the onset and offset are gradual and show a smooth slowly progressive acceleration or deceleration of the auricles. This sequence is generally associated with an abrupt "shift" in the form of the auricular complex from normal to abnormal or vice versa. For a longer or shorter period of time, and particularly during the development or recession of the arrhythmia, there may be a 1:1 ventricular response. At this time to all intents and purposes this is classical atrial tachycardia; the error of this misinterpretation

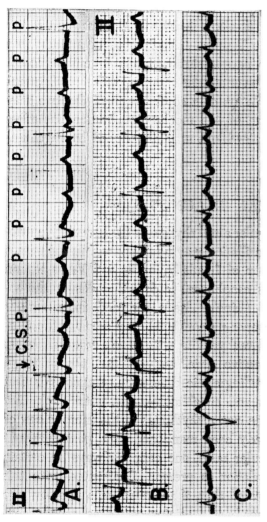

Fig. 23. *Three Examples of Atrial Tachycardia with Block.* Lead II throughout. (A) First five cycles show 1:1 conduction. Carotid sinus stimulation induces A-V block, first 2:1 then 3:1. Atria regular, atrial rate 170. Due to digitalis intoxication. (B) Atrial rate 168, ventricular rate 96. Atria show very slight irregularity and the block is variable. Here the arrhythmia was not due to digitalis and was not helped by potassium. (C) Associated with sagging RS-T segments and a single ventricular premature beat, the first indicating digitalis effect, the second, like the principal arrhythmia, reflecting digitalis intoxication. Atrial rate 210, ventricular rate 140. Atria slightly irregular. Wenckbach phenomenon with 3:2 response.

[237]

is avoided by the demonstration of atrioventricular block on carotid sinus stimulation. The block, spontaneous or induced, is usually partial (second degree). There may be a 2:1 response or a variable type of response and the Wenckebach phenomenon may be demonstrable. If alternate P deflections are lost in the QRS complexes or the T waves the existence of 2:1 response may be missed and a normal sinus mechanism misdiagnosed. Careful scrutiny of the ventricular complex or the employment of carotid sinus stimulation or a combination of the two may reveal the true nature of the mechanism. In rare instances complete atrioventricular block may be induced by vagal maneuvers.

DIFFERENTIAL DIAGNOSIS

Because of the irregular atrial rhythm or the irregular ventricular response atrial fibrillation may be simulated. In such cases meticulous examination of Leads V_1 or V_1 and V_2 or certain special leads such as esophageal leads, CR leads or the so-called Wilson leads (bipolar leads recorded from various points on the right upper precordium) may disclose the individual blips of atrial tachycardia with block when all other leads show no distinctive atrial activity. But the principal difficulty in electrocardiographic differential diagnosis is that between atrial flutter and atrial tachycardia with block. The difference between the two arrhythmias in the morphology of the baseline has already been mentioned. But, particularly at the more rapid auricular rates, one cannot always be certain whether or not undulation is present. Confronted with this problem it may be stated that, if the atrial rate is below 200 *and* the patient has not been receiving quinidine, atrial tachycardia with block is present; and if the atrial rate exceeds 250, flutter is probably the mechanism whether the auricular baseline is undulant or iso-electric. The greatest difficulty is

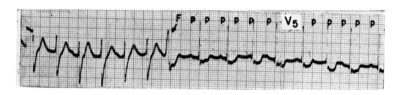

Fig. 24. Atrial tachycardia with block complicated by ventricular tachycardia. Strip shows end of bout of ventricular tachycardia, a fusion beat marking the transition. Atrial rate 180 throughout. Ventricular rate 125 during earlier portion, 115 during latter.

experienced when the auricular rate is in the twilight zone
between 200 and 250 and the baseline is iso-electric. Decision
is vital. Does the patient have atrial flutter and require that
digitalis be started, continued or increased? Or does he have
atrial tachycardia with block? And if he does have atrial tachycardia with block is it that variety which is due to digitalis
intoxication or that which is unrelated to digitalis? Faced with
this dilemma, and unable to make an electrocardiographic differentiation, the physician must now make a decision based
upon an evaluation of the clinical set-up. In the last analysis
the question is really not whether this is atrial tachycardia
with block or atrial flutter but whether or not the patient is
intoxicated with digitalis. If the patient has received actual
physical overdose of the drug, or has been the subject of a
recent insult such as acute myocardial infarction or acute cor
pulmonale which somehow makes him sensitive to previously
tolerated maintenance doses of the drug, or if he has been the
subject of such potassium-depleting procedures (see Chapter
7) as a large diuresis, chlorothiazide (Diuril) therapy, "potassium losing" nephritis, cortisone therapy, dialysis, etc.,
digitalis intoxication is possible or likely. One then takes the
tentative tack that digitalis intoxication is present and treats the
patient accordingly. If, on the contrary, one decides that digitalis intoxication is unlikely or impossible, one proceeds cautiously or boldly with digitalis. In either case, if the subsequent
course of events contradicts the original impression, or if the
patient gets worse on a selected course, one may then change
tack. In these borderline cases this trial of therapy may not
only establish the rôle of digitalis but also, from the dynamic-
electrocardiographic sequence thus induced, clarify the original electrocardiographic diagnosis.

Reference has just been made to the need for clinical judgment in doubtful instances of atrial tachycardia with block.
The same injunction holds, for that matter, in the assessment

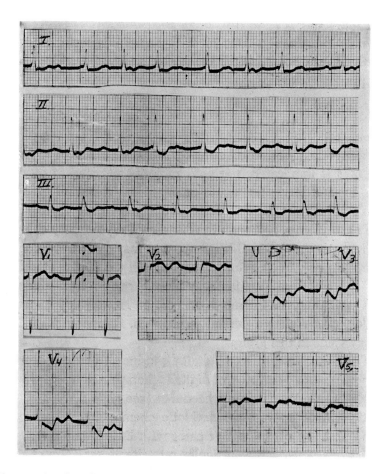

Fig. 25. *Atrial Tachycardia with Block with Potassium Depletion.* Elderly man with hypertensive heart disease on maintenance digitalis therapy. Tracings recorded immediately after large mercurial-induced diuresis. RS-T segments depressed, T waves inverted, U waves prominent. Atrial rate 170, ventricular rate 95 to 105. Reverted on omitting digitalis and giving KCl, 1 gm. t.i.d.

of all cases of atrial tachycardia with block, even where an electrocardiographic diagnosis is indubitable. With an atrial rate below 200 and the auricular baseline clearly iso-electric, the real point at issue is whether the patient is suffering from digitalis intoxication. One must therefore always consider all of the background factors mentioned in the preceding paragraph.

MANAGEMENT

Alongside these cases of atrial tachycardia with block in which digitalis is implicated, the 30% minority not due to digitalis are, by and large, not acute emergencies. Especially if they don't have heart disease, these patients are little disabled by their arrhythmia. Although the disordered rhythm may be more difficult to control in this group, one may generally proceed more leisurely in its management than in the digitalis-induced variety. Full digitalization may slow a rapid ventricular rate and quinidine, in tolerated dosage, or conceivably procaine amide, may restore a normal mechanism. Potassium is of little if any value in this group.

Treatment in the larger, digitalis-induced, group comprises two phases: (1) omission of digitalis therapy and of potassium-depleting medications or procedures (see page 165); and (2) institution of appropriate antidotic chemotherapy (see page 169). In some of the milder cases with little if any symptoms and a relatively slow ventricular rate simple cessation of digitalis therapy may be all that is required. In the course of 24 to 48 hours the patient is back in normal sinus rhythm. In patients with somewhat more severe symptoms and a moderately elevated ventricular rate, due account being taken of the status of renal function, one may give potassium by mouth. During the slowing of the auricular rate induced by potassium there is commonly a period, of variable duration, of 1:1

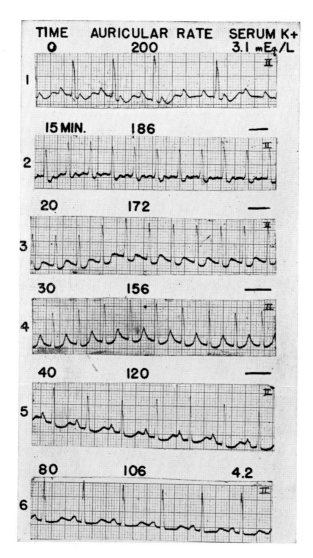

Fig. 26. *Electrocardiographic sequence during potassium therapy for atrial tachycardia with block.* The atrial rate slows progressively from 200 to 120. In strip 2 there is a 1:1 response phase which persists through strip 5. As the atria slow the ventricular rate increases: the clinical condition of the patient may deteriorate at this time. Such transient 1:1 response may also occur during the spontaneous inception and recession of the arrhythmia. A similar sequence is expected during Pronestyl therapy, a reverse chronological sequence during the development of the arrhythmia as induced by potassium extraction or digitalis overdosage. Between strips 5 and 6 the mechanism reverts to normal sinus rhythm.

[243]

response. (Fig. 23,B.) As in the quinidine treatment of atrial flutter, the ventricles may thus temporarily speed up as the auricles slow. This is apt to be alarming since the condition of the patient may actually get worse at this time. However, assuming that the atria have slowed progressively up to this point, potassium therapy must be pushed, for with further increments the ventricles will also slow and eventually a normal mechanism be restored.

Where the patient is vomiting or cannot tolerate oral potassium or where the condition of the patient seems precarious and it is anticipated that a prolonged 1:1 response phase will be poorly tolerated, potassium is given by vein rather than by mouth. This more aggressive therapy abbreviates the 1:1 phase and, with careful electrocardiographic monitoring, is actually safer than the oral route. If, at the end of the infusion of 40 mEq. of potassium, the auricles have not slowed it is unlikely that further amounts of potassium will be effective. If they have slowed but reversion has not yet occurred, more potassium is infused until normal sinus rhythm is restored. In our [1] experience at the Peter Bent Brigham Hospital this has required from 20 to 120 mEq. (average 58 mEq.).

As an alternative one may give procaine amide (Pronestyl) as described on pages 186 and 280. Where there is clear-cut clinical or laboratory evidence of potassium losses, primary reliance should be placed upon potassium supplementation. Potassium and procaine amide should be used in combination where the auricular rate is rapid and a 1:1 response phase with rapid ventricular rate is anticipated. Where the two are used together the individual requirement of each is decreased.

Sodium ethylenediamine tetraacetic acid (Na-EDTA) which binds calcium ion and thus controls digitalis intoxication has also been reported as effective in atrial tachycardia with block.[4]

REFERENCES

(1) Lown, B. and Levine, H. D.: Atrial Arrhythmias, Digitalis and Potassium. Landsberger Medical Books, New York, 1958.

(2) Lown, B., Marcus, F. and Levine, H. D.: Digitalis and atrial tachycardia with block. A year's experience. N.E.J. Med. 260: 301, 1959.

(3) Lown, B., Wyatt, N. F. and Levine, H. D.: Clinical progress, Paroxysmal atrial tachycardia with block. Circ. 21: 129, 1960.

(4) Jick, S. and Karsh, R.: The effect of calcium on chelation, cardiac arrhythmias and conduction disturbances. Am. J. Cardiol. 4: 287, 1959.

12

ATRIAL FIBRILLATION

Diagnosis

Differential Diagnosis

Management

Special Considerations

12

ATRIAL FIBRILLATION

It is only in conjunction with a rapid ventricular rate, with congestive heart failure or with embolism that atrial fibrillation may become an acute medical emergency. At its onset, atrial fibrillation may be associated with a rapid ventricular response and induce syncope, shock or the development or aggravation of congestive heart failure. Ordinarily this doesn't occur unless there is heart disease in the background. Atrial fibrillation of long duration, in the presence of advancing congestive heart failure or of certain complications such as acute pulmonary embolism or any acute infection such as pneumonia, bacterial endocarditis or myocarditis, may likewise be attended with a rapid ventricular rate.

DIAGNOSIS

When the ventricular rate is not rapid, atrial fibrillation is generally quite readily recognized both at the bedside and with the electrocardiogram. The ventricular rhythm is grossly irregular. There is not, as in flutter, an underlying dominant regularity. The ventricular rhythm has neither rhyme nor reason. It is impossible deliberately to tap in unison with the cardiac rhythm. The longer pauses which may be heard are not necessarily preceded by short pauses as one would expect when

dealing with premature beats. In uncomplicated atrial fibrillation irregular beating is not interrupted by shorter or longer
salvos of regular beating of the ventricles as it may be in
flutter. In fibrillation moreover, although there may be some
variation in the intensity of the first sound, this is never as
pronounced as in flutter. The ventricular beats may or may not
induce palpable pulses at the wrists. There may thus be a
discrepancy between the heart rate as heard at the apex and
the pulse rate as felt at the wrist. This "pulse deficit", which
is a measure of frustrate beating of the heart, is never large
when the ventricles are not rapid. The electrocardiogram shows
irregularly disposed ventricular complexes but there are no
clearcut recurrent P waves. Instead, the baseline between the
ventricular complexes may show a gross or fine, wavy undulation of varying form. (Fig. 14.) There is a variation in the time
interval between successive oscillations ("f" or fibrillation
waves) of the baseline. (Fig. 27.) Their rate varies between 350
and 600 per minute. An overzealous imagination may seize
upon some of the random meanderings of the baseline as P
waves (Fig. 27,B); this is a frequent source of diagnostic error;
true P waves are clear-cut, regular or fairly regular and should
have the same or similar form from complex to complex. In
atrial fibrillation the ventricular complexes, with some exceptions, are usually of the same form as those observed when
the patient is in normal sinus rhythm.

On the basis of the criteria just detailed the diagnosis of
atrial fibrillation is generally made quite readily. When the
ventricular rate has been slowed, as by digitalis, the detection
of this arrhythmia is somewhat more difficult. Except when
complicated by embolism, however, such a slow fibrillating
heart would hardly present as an acute emergency. When the
ventricles are very rapid the diagnosis is not easy, particularly
if this must be made from bedside observation. There may be
the same difficulty even when electrocardiograms are available.

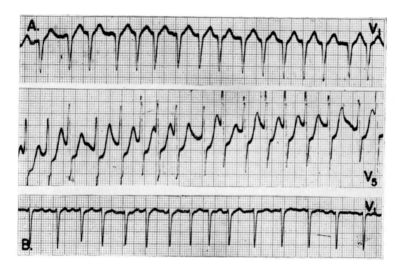

Fig. 27. *Atrial Fibrillation with Rapid Ventricular Rate.* (A) Tracings re-corded in 58-year-old man with hypertensive and coronary heart disease. P waves and fibrillation waves not identified. Ventricular rate as high as 170. Pronounced RS-T segment depression probably related to subendocardial ischemia. The peaking of the latter part of the T waves could erroneously be attributed to P waves but this peaking is clearly related to the preceding, not the succeeding, ventricular complex and is therefore part of the T wave. On digitalis patient reverted to normal rhythm later that day. (B) Tracings re-corded in a 48-year-old bartender with cirrhosis of the liver in severe con-gestive heart failure. Fibrillation ("f") waves are visible, some simulating normal P waves (e.g. those before the 2nd, 3rd, 7th, 8th and 14th ventricular com-plex). Ventricular rate as high as 164. Digitalis by mouth or vein ineffective. Slowed to 90 on large doses of thiamin.

With a fast heart rate it is not quite so easy to appreciate the variability in cycle length, the lack of a dominant regularity, the less pronounced variations in the first sound and the fact that the longer pauses are not preceded by shorter pauses. And in the electrocardiogram when one beat follows tumultuously after another it may be difficult to define the exact appearance of the baseline. (Fig. 27,A.) If the patient has been receiving digitalis there may be, for shorter or longer periods, a regular ventricular rhythm but, if long enough strips are examined, the slight irregularity will generally be detected.

Atrial fibrillation may at times be associated with a persistent regularity of the ventricles. This is the result of complicating complete heart block or, more commonly, of nodal tachycardia, and generally denotes digitalis intoxication.

DIFFERENTIAL DIAGNOSIS

Atrial fibrillation is to be distinguished from atrial premature beats, from atrial flutter, from atrial tachycardia with block and from ventricular tachycardia. Where atrial premature beats are rare or occasional the problem is not a difficult one. But where they are frequent and where the "timetable" of the sino-auricular node is upset by the penetration of some of the premature beats into the sinus node, the differentiation is more difficult. The point has already been made that with atrial premature beats a long pause is necessarily preceded by a quick beat; the pause is, to a greater or lesser extent, compensatory. In uncomplicated atrial fibrillation long pauses are not necessarily preceded by short pauses. With atrial premature beats there are no characteristic fibrillation waves. Each early ventricular complex is preceded by a P wave. This may resemble the normal P wave or have a different contour. It has often to be suspected by the very slightest deformity in the contour of the T wave of the preceding ventricular complex, sometimes by a mere exaggeration in its height. The ventricular complex may have the same configuration as the normally conducted beats but when very premature the succeeding ventricular complexes may be aberrant and resemble ventricular premature beats.

The differentiation between atrial flutter and atrial fibrillation is described on pages 223 and 224. The importance of this distinction lies not in immediate treatment; it is quite similar in either case. But in the matter of deciding to just what lengths one would be willing to go in order to accomplish reversion to normal sinus rhythm, it is quite important to have made the distinction. Because of the extreme lability of the heart rate in flutter the patient is generally in a more precarious condition than he would be in fibrillation. Furthermore there is much less risk of embolization on attempting reversion in flutter than there is in fibrillation. All other things being equal, therefore, one is much more eager to undertake reversion in patients with flutter. As we shall see, however, there will be occasional patients with atrial fibrillation and persistently rapid ventricular rate, who are doing badly, in whom it will be worthwhile to attempt reversion.

The differentiation between atrial fibrillation and atrial tachycardia with block is made by the electrocardiogram. The decisive feature in atrial tachycardia with block is the regularly or slightly irregularly recurring P waves occurring at a rate generally between 150 and 200, but occasionally as fast as 250. These waves are separated by an iso-electric baseline. In fibrillation P waves are not recognized and the baseline shows a fine or coarse irregular undulation.

Atrial fibrillation associated with intraventricular block (e.g. bundle branch block) (Fig. 31) may simulate tachycardia of the ventricles. The impulses arise in the auricles and irregularly filter down into the ventricles; at the same time the QRS complexes are prolonged as a result of the intraventricular block.

This block may have been demonstrated previously, or prove to be present subsequently, during normal sinus rhythm. Similar spreading out of the ventricular complexes may be seen in the absence of true intraventricular block when an ectopic rhythm arises in the ventricle and activates the ventricle eccentrically (ventricular tachycardia). How is one to decide whether the impulse arises in the fibrillating atria and is conducted aberrantly into the ventricles (intraventricular block) or arises ectopically in the ventricle? The ventricular rhythm is irregular in atrial fibrillation. It is regular in about half of the cases of ventricular tachycardia, slightly irregular in the other half. But there is often a difference between the irregularity in atrial fibrillation and that in ventricular tachycardia. As a general rule, the irregularity of the ventricles in atrial fibrillation is readily apparent on first listening. It doesn't require that degree of close attention which is so necessary in dealing with paroxysmal ventricular tachycardia, to decide that the ventricular rhythm really is slightly irregular. This is probably due in part to the average slower rate of the ventricles in atrial fibrillation than in ventricular tachycardia and the easier detection of arrhythmia when the heart is slow than when it is rapid. It may also be related to a greater inherent tendency to regularity in ventricular tachycardia than in atrial fibrillation, even at the same heart rate. Considerations already enumerated (page 224) differentiating between atrial flutter with intraventricular block, on the one hand, and ventricular tachycardia on the other, are also applicable in the differentiation between atrial fibrillation with intraventricular block and ventricular tachycardia.

The variations in the intensity of the first heart sound are generally much more striking in paroxysmal ventricular tachycardia than in atrial fibrillation. Carotid sinus stimulation has no effect whatever upon the rhythm or rate of the ventricles in paroxymsal ventricular tachycardia. In atrial fibrillation this procedure may slow the ventricular rate while the ventricular rhythm remains grossly irregular.

MANAGEMENT

Treatment consists of optimal digitalization. The speed and route of digitalization depends, as always, upon the urgency of the clinical situation. This may be accomplished with an oral preparation as described on page 226. Where this is truly a grave emergency, an intravenous injection should be given. The particular preparation used will depend in large part upon the experience of the physician. He should be familiar with the use of one intravenous preparation. In a patient who has received no digitalis during the previous two or three weeks 1.0 mgm. of Digoxin may be given by vein as the initial dose followed by 0.25 mgm. every two hours until a therapeutic effect has been achieved or a total dose of 1.5 mgm. has been given.[1] An alternative would be Cedilanid 0.8 mgm. by vein followed by 0.4 mgm. every two hours as necessary. If the patient has received digitalis previously or if the patient's state of digitalization is unknown, one may give 0.25 to 0.5 mgm. of Digoxin as the initial dose and repeat 0.25 mgm. at 2 to 4-hourly intervals. Once the rate has been slowed, digitalization may be maintained with an oral preparation such as digitalis leaf, 0.1 gm. daily or Digoxin 0.5 mgm. daily, the exact maintenance dose to be determined by trial and error. Incredibly large amounts of digitalis may often be required to slow the ventricular rate of a patient who has already, to all intents and purposes, been adequately digitalized and who develops atrial fibrillation with a rapid ventricular rate or whose heart has been fibrillating with a slow ventricular rate and now, for one reason or another, develops a faster heart rate. It is surprising, too, how often, in addition to slowing the ventricular rate, digitalization is actually followed by reversion to normal sinus rhythm, particularly if the fibrillation is of recent onset.

Where an extremely rapid effect is considered imperative Ouabain (Strophanthin G) should be given by vein. The initial dose is 0.5 mgm. Its effect is observed within 5 to 15 minutes. Maximal effect is obvious in from ½ to 2 hours.[2] Increments of 0.1 mgm. may be given in a half-hour and repeated every hour until a therapeutic effect has been achieved but the total dose should not exceed 1.0 mgm. within a 24-hour period.

SPECIAL CONSIDERATIONS

In many cases, paroxysms of atrial fibrillation are an emergency only in the minds of the patient's family. Apart from the rapid heart action he may appear quite well. In these cases oral digitalization may be all that is necessary. In rare instances alcohol may precipitate atrial fibrillation. This disappears when the alcohol is metabolized. There are some patients in congestive heart failure with enlarged fibrillating hearts who present no evidence whatever of heart disease. They are not and have never been hypertensive. They have never had rheumatic fever or an allied disorder and physical examination shows none of the stigmata of rheumatic valvular disease. They have never had angina pectoris and laboratory and physical examination discloses no evidence for myocardial infarction. This particular subgroup should be sought out deliberately for it represents a very special indication for reversion. On restoration to normal sinus rhythm these patients may lose all evidence of cardiac impairment and become perfectly normal individuals. It is a rare but exceedingly gratifying experience to find such a patient.

It is well recognized that patients with atrial fibrillation due to thyrotoxicosis are generally quite unresponsive to digitalis therapy. At times it seems impossible to slow their ventricles. But there are a few in whom larger doses will accomplish ventricular slowing when ordinary doses have been ineffective. The important point is that this very refractoriness to digitalis should alert the physician to the diagnosis of hyperthyroidism in the first place. The major therapeutic indication is not to slow the heart but to treat the underlying thyrotoxic state. Generally one should not waste time in trying to restore normal rhythm before definitive antithyroid therapy is given, be it radio-active iodine therapy, subtotal thyroidectomy or propyl-thiouracil. Two or three weeks after successful medical or surgical treatment, reversion may be undertaken if it has not already occurred spontaneously. This is generally a leisurely process with prompt response to relatively small doses of quinidine. The same considerations apply to patients with rheumatic valvular heart disease who are to be subjected to mitral valvuloplasty. One should not waste time reverting them to normal sinus rhythm preoperatively. The attempt is not always successful and even if reversion is accomplished, these patients are prone to re-develop this arrhythmia during or after surgery. It is wiser to wait until late in the post-operative period or even later before reversion is attempted.

Atrial fibrillation is not uncommon as a complication of acute myocardial infarction. Frequently it is a transient phenomenon which disappears spontaneously in a few hours. The danger of digitalis inducing toxic rhythms is enhanced in the presence of myocardial infarction. It seems worth-while therefore, under these circumstances, to withhold digitalis therapy until it seems obvious that spontaneous reversion will not occur or unless the condition of the patient deteriorates.

Atrial fibrillation occasionally develops acutely during a surgical operation. The subcutaneous injection of 1 or 2 mgms. of Prostigmine may then promptly and adequately slow the ventricles so that the surgeon may proceed with the operation. The arrhythmia may then be dealt with definitively in a more leisurely fashion after the operation. Where Prostigmine is ineffective, resort may be had to an intravenous digitalis preparation.

Atrial fibrillation, occurring during active rheumatic carditis, responds poorly to digitalis or quinidine. It is only when specific treatment such as salicylate or cortisone is given that the arrhythmia is brought under control. Atrial fibrillation associated with chronic rheumatic valvular heart disease may present a very special problem in management, that of recurrent embolism. Mitral valvuloplasty or long-term anticoagulant therapy might then be appropriate. Embolism is an infrequent consequence of atrial fibrillation in thyrotoxic, hypertensive or coronary heart disease.

For well over a quarter of a century there has been a running controversy regarding the risk of dislodging thrombi from the atrium and inducing peripheral or pulmonary embolism upon reversion of atrial fibrillation to normal sinus rhythm with quinidine. The point of view adopted by a particular authority apparently depends upon his individual experience. I cannot help but be impressed from my own practice that the danger is a very real one. In many fatal instances of embolism following reversion the atria are found at post-mortem examination to be clear of thrombi. It seems reasonable therefore to suspect that many of these emboli are dislodged from auricular thrombi which form, then and there, at the instant of reversion. The evidence is not altogether convincing but many authorities prefer to administer anticoagulant therapy before starting quinidine therapy for reversion. There is some difference of opinion on just how this should be accomplished. Some prefer to maintain the patient within the optimal anticoagulant range for a week or so before starting quinidine. Others are content to start quinidine once the optimal range is attained. My own experience has been with dicumarol used in this way. I know of no reason why heparin or any other anticoagulant should not be equally effective as dicumarol. It appears to be unnecessary to give anticoagulants before attempting reversion after successful valvuloplasty. Here presumably the stasis or eddy currents existing behind the stenosed mitral valve have been eliminated by the operation and the new hemodynamic situation is not conducive to intra-atrial thrombosis.

It is only rarely that quinidine is called upon as an emergency medication in the treatment of atrial fibrillation. It is generally used in a more leisurely fashion when it is felt that there would be greater advantage to the patient if his heart were in normal sinus rhythm than in perpetual atrial fibrillation. There are some circumstances however where the drug must be considered for emergency use. If the patient with atrial fibrillation with rapid heart rate and congestive heart failure fails to slow on what appears to be optimal digitalis dosage, and the clinician feels assured that this is not the result of non-absorption of digitalis, a deliberate and desperate attempt should be make to revert the heart to normal sinus rhythm with quinidine despite the rapid heart rate. The details of this procedure are given on page 279 in the discussion of ventricular tachycardia. This effort is ordinarily not as successful as the attempt to revert atrial fibrillation when the rate has already been slowed by digitalis.

The management of nodal tachycardia or complete heart block complicating atrial fibrillation is considered under digitalis toxicity (page 185).

REFERENCES

(1) Levine, H. D. and Levine, S. A.: The management of cardiac emergencies. Med. Clin. No. Am. p. 965, July 1953. (Nationwide issue).

(2) Master, A. M., Moser, M. and Jaffe, H. L.: Cardiac Emergencies and Heart Failure. Lea and Febiger, Philadelphia, 1955. p. 22.

13

PAROXYSMAL VENTRICULAR TACHYCARDIA

Electrocardiographic Diagnosis

Differential Diagnosis

Treatment

CHAPTER

13

PAROXYSMAL VENTRICULAR

TACHYCARDIA

Tachycardia of the ventricles is one of the most critical of the arrhythmias. In the hierarchy of ectopic ventricular disturbances it is a step above ventricular premature beats and the forerunner of ventricular fibrillation. In man the latter is probably generally pre-terminal. In the overwhelming majority, ventricular tachycardia occurs in patients with heart disease. It is of the utmost importance that this condition be recognized as such since prompt treatment can be lifesaving. Its gravity is highlighted by the fact that even in some of the few instances where it has developed in patients without heart disease it has been the immediate cause of death. In about three-fourths of cases it occurs in patients with coronary artery disease [1] either during an episode of acute coronary thrombosis or in patients who have survived an acute attack of myocardial infarction or who have coronary artery disease as judged by other evidence. As a complication of acute myocardial infarction this arrhythmia represents an added threat to the survival of the patient. Ventricular tachycardia may also occur in patients with rheumatic heart disease, particularly those in congestive heart failure receiving digitalis. Paroxysmal ventricular tachycardia may develop as a toxic manifestation of therapy with quinidine or procaine amide. It may arise in the more advanced phases of potassium intoxication. It occurs rarely in severe thyrotoxicosis. Not uncommonly it develops in patients with complete heart block; in these individuals and in congenital heart disease this tachycardia, rather than excessive slowing or asystole of the ventricles may be the cause of the syncopal attacks. For a time it was considered that the Wolff-Parkinson-White syndrome may be complicated by paroxysmal ventricular tachycardia; in most of the reported instances, however, the tracings published as ventricular tachycardia seem more like those of supraventricular arrhythmias, atrial fibrillation [2] or flutter, the ventricular complexes being those characterizing the "anomalous" in contradistinction to the "normal" type of ventricular excitation seen in this syndrome. In about 10 or 15% of cases no cardiac abnormality is discovered on reversion to normal rhythm; in this particular group the outlook is excellent once reversion has been achieved.

An observed paroxysm is clearly abrupt in onset and offset and the patient is generally conscious of its inception. Apparently the patient's awareness of the arrhythmia depends upon his previous condition. If he has been quite well and up and about, his condition at the onset of the arrhythmia naturally stands in marked contrast to his previous state of health and he is quite aware of the change. On the other hand I have discovered the tachycardia during routine rounds when patients with acute myocardial infarction have reported that they were feeling quite well. In such a case, since the patient has not recognized this new development, his physician may not know just how long it had lasted. The attack might have started 12 hours or five minutes previously. Other individuals, on the other hand, might be thrown rapidly into collapse or congestive failure at the onset of their paroxysm. Some might become dizzy or even lose consciousness. Indeed, as we have seen, syncope may develop at the onset of paroxysmal rapid heart action of any type; this includes paroxysmal ventricular tachycardia no matter what its underlying etiology. Chest pain resembling that of angina pectoris or coronary thrombosis may also occur at the onset of paroxysmal ventricular tachycardia. The rate of the heart varies from about 140 to 240, rarely higher. In about half of the cases the rhythm is quite regular. In the other half close attention will show that it is very slightly but definitely irregular. It may, in fact, be necessary to listen for some time before this irregularity is appreciated. The variations in cycle length seem to be much more subtle than those occurring, for example, in atrial fibrillation at a comparable ventricular rate. (Fig. 27.) Much more important in a diagnostic way is the audible variation in the intensity of the first heart sound (Fig. 28) in an attack.[3,4,5] This derives from the fact that ventricular tachycardia is generally a dissociated rhythm; the atria are driven by a sinus pacemaker and the ventricles by a ventricular pacemaker. It is the changing relationship between atrial and ventricular contraction which accounts for the changing loudness of the first sound. In those rare instances of paroxysmal ventricular tachycardia in which the ventricles are driving the auricles regularly (1:1 retrograde atrial activation) or where the atria are fibrillating, a change in the intensity of S_1 will not be observed. Stimulation of the carotid sinus has no effect whatever upon the ventricular mechanism in ventricular tachycardia. Observation of the jugular pulse [6,7] may at times be helpful in this diagnosis. One may see an extra forceful flick to the jugular pulse due to closer coincidence of atrial and ventricular contraction. At other times it may be observed that the rate of pulsation of the jugular vein is slower than the ventricular rate as heard at the apex.

I have seen one instance of ventricular tachycardia in which the apparent heart rate was just one half of the true rate. This is one of three such cases mentioned by Armbrust and Levine.[1]

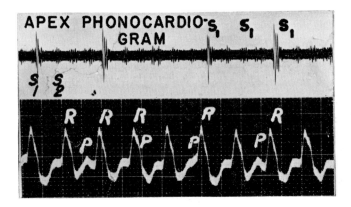

Fig. 28. *Variation in intensity of first sound in paroxysmal ventricular tachy-cardia*. Upper trace shows apical phonocardiogram, lower trace standard Lead II. The ventricular complexes are broad, bizarre and of variable contour. Independent atrial activity.

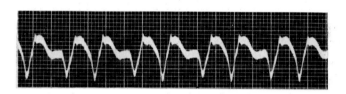

Fig. 29. *Normal sinus rhythm* (rate 83) *simulated by paroxysmal ventricular tachycardia with alternation in cycle length.* (Ventricular rate 165). A second sound was heard in neither the short nor the long cycle. The sound following the long pause seemed to be S_1, that following the short pause S_2.

This resulted from the fact that in this patient there was at times an alternation in cycle length (Fig. 29). Only one heart sound was audible in each cycle and the sound of one cycle was different from that of the next. Thus the sound of one cycle was considered to be first sound, and that of the next cycle the second sound of a single cycle. It is easy to see how the true rate and its significance could have been missed in the first place, or how, even if it were already known that ventricular tachycardia was present, this phenomenon could have been misinterpreted as signalling reversion.

Strictly speaking the findings just described may be detected in other forms of atrioventricular dissociation with a nodal rather than a ventricular focus setting the ventricular pace. It is always desirable to record an electrocardiogram. It may settle this point but will not always be decisive. It may be taken as a reliable first approximation, however, that *the development of a heart rate exceeding 150 with a slightly irregular rhythm and associated with changes in the loudness of the first sound, in an individual with coronary artery disease, is due to tachycardia of the ventricle until proven otherwise.*

ELECTROCARDIOGRAPHIC DIAGNOSIS

A presumptive electrocardiographic diagnosis of paroxysmal ventricular tachycardia may be made on the basis of three features. The first of these is a broadened bizarre ventricular complex. The widened QRS complex expresses the ectopic origin and aberrant spread of ventricular activation. The second feature is the somewhat variable appearance of the complex. This is the result of atrioventricular dissociation. The P waves are often difficult to recognize but when identifiable occur clearly at a different rate than the ventricular complexes. Because of the changing relationships between auricular and ventricular activation the P waves are inscribed at different points in the ventricular complexes of successive cycles. In one cycle it might form a slur on the ascending limb, in the next it might occur at the apex, and in the next it might deform the downstroke of the R wave. When there is retrograde activation of the atria the form of the ventricular complex will not change. The ventricular rhythm may be regular or slightly irregular. The latter is due either to a varying block about the ventricular pacemaker or to what Katz and Pick have been pleased to call "variability in the exaltation" of the ventricular pacemaker.[8] The third and final feature is the failure of this mechanism to be influenced by carotid sinus stimulation or other vagal maneuvers; this procedure may slow the atrial rhythm when the latter is decipherable. At times paroxysmal tachycardia may be considered as probably ventricular in origin if the contour of the QRS complex of isolated ventricular premature beats which follow an attack is identical with or very similar to that of the paroxysm.

The objection can be raised that even if all the above enumerated criteria are satisfied it is still possible that one is not dealing with ventricular tachycardia. In atrioventricular dissociation the auricles may be driven by the sinus node and the ventricles not by a ventricular pacemaker but by the atrioventricular node. If intraventricular block is present the ventricular complexes would be bizarre and prolonged and since atrioventricular dissociation is present the ventricular complexes would display a variable form. These considerations would be valid whether or not abnormal ventricular complexes have been demonstrated during normal rhythm for aberrant ventricular conduction may be a function of the heart rate. Thus many alleged instances of ventricular tachycardia are actually nodal tachycardia with intraventricular block. Much more often than not it is impossible to be certain which of these two mechanisms is present. In this quandary two findings may be quite helpful in making a decision. The first of these

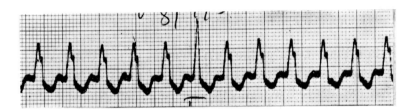

Fig. 30. A single *normal ventricular complex within a bout of ventricular tachy-cardia.* This is not rate-conditioned intraventricular block for this beat is of normal duration without change in rate. This is a "captured" ventricular beat. By exclusion the remaining beats are not conducted over the main auriculo-ventricular stem and must be ectopic in origin.

is the finding of a normal ventricular complex (Fig. 30) during a bout of tachycardia in which the remaining complexes
are bizarre.[8] This is due to the fact that during atrioventricular
dissociation—in contrast to atrioventricular *block*—atrioventricular conduction is still possible. Under these circumstances
an atrial beat may be conducted to the ventricles at a moment
when they have recovered from their refractory phase. The
ventricle is then "captured." The fact that the ventricular complex is now normal or at least is identical with the usual complexes of the same lead during normal rhythm, shows that a
beat conducted from the atria over the usual atrioventricular
pathways is capable of inducing normal complexes. Since the
remaining complexes of the paroxysm are abnormal and the
ventricular rate has not changed, these beats could not have
passed through the atrioventricular node. By exclusion then
the abnormal complexes must have arisen "off the beaten path"
and the mechanism must be paroxysmal ventricular tachycardia. Even better evidence for this diagnosis would be the
detection during a bout of tachycardia with abnormal ventricular complexes of fusion ventricular complexes,[9] that is, complexes which are clearly a blend of the normal or indigenous
complexes for that lead and those characterizing the paroxysm
(Fig. 24). It must then be reasoned that at least one of these
fusing impulses has to arise below the level of the bifurcation
of the atrioventricular bundle to blend in the ventricles with
the impulses conducted from the atria. By exclusion the mechanism must be ventricular and not nodal tachycardia.

DIFFERENTIAL DIAGNOSIS

Paroxysmal ventricular tachycardia may be confused clinically with various supraventricular arrhythmias, (atrial fibrillation, atrial flutter, classical paroxysmal atrial tachycardia,
atrial tachycardia with block and paroxysmal nodal tachy-

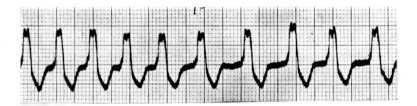

Fig. 31. *Atrial fibrillation with left bundle branch block.* On superficial examination this resembles paroxysmal ventricular tachycardia but the variation in cycle length is much more pronounced than is observed in that disturbance.

cardia). And any of these arrhythmias when associated with intraventricular block may simulate ventricular tachycardia electrocardiographically. As in dealing with puzzling arrhythmias in general a test of the effect of carotid sinus stimulation is mandatory. From both the bedside and electrocardiographic standpoint it may demonstrate a manner of response quite inconsistent with ventricular tachycardia, namely, cessation of the attack in paroxysmal atrial or nodal tachycardia, or transient slowing of the ventricles in atrial fibrillation or flutter, or atrial tachycardia with block. And where the question of supraventricular tachycardia with intraventricular block is being considered this procedure may disclose two further bits of information. When the rate of the ventricles is sufficiently slowed by this maneuver a characteristic contour of the basline, either that of atrial fibrillation or flutter or atrial tachycardia with block, may be uncovered. Furthermore, during the slowed phase a normal or relatively normal configuration of the ventricular complex may be produced (Fig. 32,A). From this one may conclude that the widened ventricular complexes observed in the paroxysm are a function of the heart rate and not a feature of the mechanism *per se*.

The differentiation of ventricular tachycardia from atrial flutter is described on page 224, from atrial fibrillation on page 253, from paroxysmal atrial or nodal tachycardia on page 202. In some cases of nodal tachycardia with apparent retrograde atrial activation, it may be difficult to decide whether a deflection contiguous to the QRS complex is a P wave or actually part of the QRS complex. The accompanying tracings (Fig. 33) are continuous recordings made in a patient with rheumatic heart disease and atrial fibrillation who developed ventricular tachycardia as a complication of digitalis overdosage. The ventricular tachycardia was interrupted by a more rapid and almost perfectly regular rhythm with ventricular

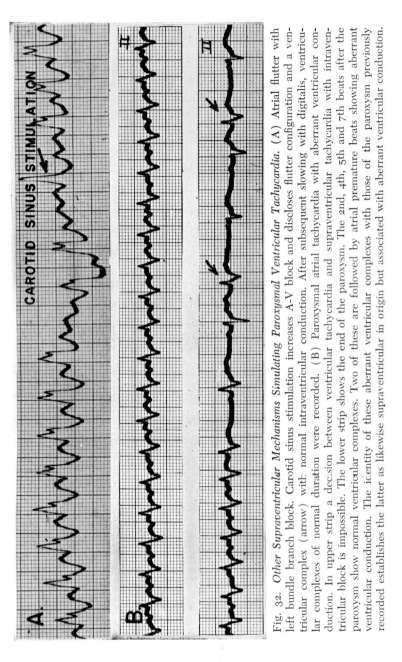

Fig. 32. *Other Supraventricular Mechanisms Simulating Paroxysmal Ventricular Tachycardia.* (A) Atrial flutter with left bundle branch block. Carotid sinus stimulation increases A-V block and discloses flutter configuration and a ventricular complex (arrow) with normal intraventricular conduction. After subsequent slowing with digitalis, ventricular complexes of normal duration were recorded. (B) Paroxysmal atrial tachycardia with aberrant ventricular conduction. In upper strip a decision between ventricular tachycardia and supraventricular tachycardia with intraventricular block is impossible. The lower strip shows the end of the paroxysm. The 2nd, 4th, 5th and 7th beats after the paroxysm show normal ventricular complexes. Two of these are followed by atrial premature beats showing aberrant ventricular conduction. The identity of these aberrant ventricular complexes with those of the paroxysm previously recorded establishes the latter as likewise supraventricular in origin but associated with aberrant ventricular conduction.

[274]

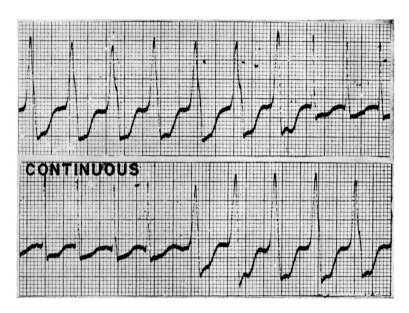

Fig. 33. Interrupted bout of ventricular tachycardia. (Continous strips.) During this rhythm the ventricular rate was 136. The interrupting mechanism is almost perfectly regular at a rate of 170 and probably represents nodal tachycardia. Atrial fibrillation was known to be in the background. This unusual tracing illustrates the inherently faster rate of the atrio-ventricular node than of the ectopic ventricular focus under identical circumstances.

complexes of normal duration. The sandwiched rhythm represents atrial fibrillation complicated by nodal tachycardia. That the inherent rate of the node is faster than that of the ventricles is demonstrated by the differences in rate during the two mechanisms, 162 during nodal tachycardia, 136 during ventricular tachycardia. It is also obvious that the bizarre complexes seen during the slower mechanism is not the effect of intraventricular block or of rate-conditioned aberrant ventricular conduction for the complexes are shorter at the faster rate. Generally the decision between ventricular tachycardia and intraventricular block complicating atrial or nodal tachycardia is much more difficult than in this case. A critical re-examination of many tracings originally interpreted as ventricular tachycardia has demonstrated many of these diagnoses to be questionable or incorrect. This may account for some of the reported successes with digitalis in alleged paroxysmal ventricular tachycardia.

I have seen only one patient in whom the differential diagnosis between ventricular tachycardia and atrial tachycardia with block had to be considered. In this individual there was a slurring of the QRS complex during the 1:1 response phase due to intraventricular block, to superimposition of the P wave on the QRS complex or to both of these causes. This phenomenon was present during only a portion of one strip and the appearance of the remainder of the tracing made the diagnosis quite clear.

ALTERNATING BIDIRECTIONAL VENTRICULAR TACHYCARDIA

Ventricular tachycardia may be a manifestation of digitalis toxicity. There is a rare sub-type of ventricular tachycardia which is practically pathognomonic of digitalis poisoning. This is alternating bidirectional ventricular tachycardia. This condi-

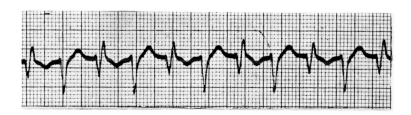

Fig. 34. *Alternating bidirectional ventricular tachycardia* developing in an 80-year-old man with coronary artery disease during digitalization. Patients with this disturbance rarely recover.

tion occurs in very diseased hearts and carries an extremely grave prognosis. The rhythm is regular and the ventricular complexes of two bizarre types, alternating one with the other. Often the main QRS complex will be upward in one complex, and downward in the next. (Fig. 34.) This is not to be confused with a condition in which the rhythm is regular and complexes of normal duration alternate with widened bizarre complexes; this is more likely to represent partial (2:1) bundle branch block. It is felt that tachycardia with alternation in cycle length [10] as well as in the form of the ventricular complexes should be regarded in the same light as that with a regular rhythm. In view of the occasional report of abolition of this disturbance by vagal maneuvers there is some question whether these may be supraventricular rather than ventricular in origin.[11,12]

TREATMENT

When the diagnosis of paroxysmal ventricular tachycardia is indubitable, therapy in general narrows down to quinidine or procaine amide (Pronestyl) given orally or parenterally. Although the use of the latter is becoming more widespread, quinidine remains the drug of choice. When the arrhythmia is first discovered it is often justifiable for a time to withhold any form of treatment if the condition of the patient seems reasonably good. In a few cases the rhythm will revert spontaneously to a normal mechanism. Such a happy turn of events is unusual. After deciding that such reversion is unlikely to occur, and assuming that the patient is in good shape, it is recommended that quinidine be given by mouth in progressively increasing doses in the pattern described in connection with atrial flutter on page 227 except that in ventricular tachycardia digitalis is not given. Even as much as 2.0 grams of quinidine may be given in a single dose in desperate cases. If this dose or the highest tolerated dose is ineffective, a subcutaneous injection of 0.5 to 2.0 mgm. of atropine, given a half hour or so after the last dose of quinidine, may be followed by reversion.[13,14] If the use of quinidine is ineffective procaine amide may be tried by mouth. If the tachycardia developed as a complication of acute coronary thrombosis the patient, once the arrhythmia has been abolished, should be maintained on oral quinidine 0.2 to 0.4 gram three or four times daily "around the clock." If the tachycardia has developed under other circumstances the question of whether maintenance quinidine should be undertaken must be decided on the merits of the case. If at the outset or sometime during the unsuccessful effort to revert the rhythm with oral medication, the patient's condition deteriorates in one way or another, as by the development of shock, congestive heart failure or recurrent chest pain, resort must be had to parenteral therapy. Many authorities prefer the intramuscular over the intravenous route, principally on the basis of its lesser tendency to produce hypotension. My experience and preference has been with the intravenous route. Among other considerations, its effect may be abbreviated by discontinuing the infusion the instant reversion has occurred whereas one may overshoot the mark with an intramuscular injection. When the latter route is used one may give 0.6 gram of the lactate, hydrochloride, gluconate or sulfate.

For intravenous use one dissolves the contents of an ampoule (0.6 gram) of quinidine sulfate, lactate or hydrochloride in 500 cc. of dextrose in water and infuses this by vein over the course of two hours. Frequent observations should be made of the blood pressure. It is generally not necessary to abandon intravenous quinidine altogether because of a hypotensive reaction. If a profound fall in blood pressure follows, the rate of infusion should be slowed. At the same time supplements of vaso-pressor amines may be administered to bring the pressure back to respectable levels.[15] The procedure should also be monitored by the use of a cardioscope or, preferably with a direct recording electrocardiogram. The latter should be running, but not necessarily recording, during the entire infusion. The infusion should be discontinued the moment reversion occurs. Maintenance oral quinidine therapy may then be instituted. If this treatment has been ineffective the subcutaneous injection of atropine may be tried within an hour of the end of the infusion. If still ineffective one may repeat the course with 0.6 or 1.2 gram of quinidine. Although it is safest to give quinidine diluted in the manner just described, there will be rare situations of desperation where it will be justified slowly to infuse the undiluted contents of an ampoule in a 5 or 10 cc. syringe. Again the blood pressure level should be carefully followed during this procedure. If quinidine is not available quinine will do. I recall one Australian sergeant who was a pedigreed reactor to the contents of one half vial of quinine (9 grains to the vial). Each of a succession of "detached" American medical officers, at a time when quinidine was not at hand, had many experiences in thus stopping his numerous bouts of ventricular tachycardia.

If quinidine is ineffective one may try procaine amide.[16] This is available in 10 cc. vials each containing one gram. This is ininjected undiluted at a rate no faster than 1 cc. per minute, discontinuing the injection the instant reversion occurs. Procaine amide may also be given diluted in large volume infusions;[17] it is my impression that it is more effective when given undiluted, safer when diluted. As with quinidine this infusion should be monitored by recordings of blood pressure and electrocardiograms. I have seen occasional instances where a second or a third gram has terminated ventricular tachycardia when smaller doses were ineffective.

The recording of frequent electrocardiograms during the course of oral or intravenous therapy with quinidine or procaine amide is not merely advisable; it is imperative.

[280]

Progressive slowing of the ventricular rate down into the "normal" range may occur though the abnormal mechanism persists. Such slowing is probably all well and good for it seems reasonable that the patient is better off with a slower than a more rapid rate. But if therapy is interrupted at this stage there is merely a progressive return of the rate to the pre-treatment level. One of the reasons for electrocardiographic control, then, is to determine that reversion to a normal mechanism has actually taken place. This is not always easy to establish during quinidine or procaine amide therapy for even when a normal mechanism is achieved the ventricular complex may be quite different in appearance from that before the paroxysm. Intraventricular block and co-incident RS-T segment and T wave changes may persist for two or three days as a pure consequence of treatment with these drugs. The post-treatment tracing may further differ from the pre-treatment electrocardiogram because it is recorded later in the course of the acute myocardial infarction which was complicated by the development of ventricular tachycardia. The sequential changes which were destined to develop at that time must inevitably appear. And finally changes in the RS-T segment and T wave, denoting myocardial ischemia and consequent upon the tachycardia per se, may persist for days or weeks. This is the so-called "post-tachycardia" syndrome and may occur in the absence of any evidence for fresh infarction. This is an important point to remember for many patients have chest pain, fever, leucocytosis, fall in blood pressure and electrocardiographic changes of this type as a consequence purely of the paroxysm of tachycardia and have been erroneously considered as having suffered a fresh myocardial infarction.

Another equally important reason for frequent electrocardiograms is to detect evidence of toxicity from quinidine or procaine amide not otherwise available. There is some difference of opinion regarding the relative toxicity of these substances but their toxic effects should be regarded as essentially similar. Each has the pharmacological effect of slowing intraventricular conduction. Although the opinion is held that this is an undesirable effect of these drugs, which tends to perpetuate rather than abolish this arrhythmia, some degree of prolongation of the QRS complex is commonly observed in patients who eventually are reverted to normal sinus rhythm with either drug. Just where the dividing line is between "safe" and "toxic" prolongation of the QRS complex is difficult to define. Arbitrary statements have been made of 25% and, later, 50% allowable increase in QRS duration but this is purely empirical and relative. When the alternative to discontinuing the drug is the persistence of the very arrhythmia which is threatening the life of the patient, it may be justifiable to increase the dosage even when such marked intraventricular block is present. Be it noted, however, that one does not lightly undertake therapy with either of these drugs in the first place.

Thus ventricular tachycardia may be treated successfully with either quinidine or procaine amide. By contrast there are some individuals in whom this disturbance develops as a toxic manifestation of either of these substances (Fig. 35), as, for example, in the treatment of supraventricular arrhythmias. In this event the precipitating drug must be discontinued forthwith.

If the patient had had permanent atrial fibrillation before the onset of the paroxysm of ventricular tachycardia he might be found, following abolition of the tachycardia, to have developed pure or impure atrial flutter. (Fig. 35,A.) This is the effect of quinidine upon the auricular mechanism; generally during the course of a day or two the atrial mechanism returns to fibrillation. Following reversion to normal sinus rhythm with quinidine the P waves may likewise be broadened, in rare cases even suggesting "mitral" P waves. This is the effect of quinidine

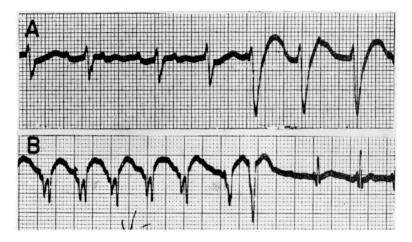

Fig. 35. *Ventricular tachycardia from drug toxicity.* (A) Paroxysm complicating quinidine therapy for atrial fibrillation. When these tracings were recorded the auricular mechanism had been changed from fibrillation to flutter (flutter rate 156). Such slow flutter rates are not uncommon after quinidine therapy. (B) Termination of bout of ventricular tachycardia complicating procaine amide therapy in patient with atrial fibrillation.

upon intra-auricular conduction. In this instance it is wise to repeat the tracings after a few days before suggesting on this basis that mitral valve disease may be present.

During the course of treatment with quinidine the patient may develop any of the symptoms of cinchonism and will often implore the physician to discontinue the treatment because of weakness, dizziness, lassitude, ringing in the ears, blurring of vision, diminished hearing or deafness, or a sense of unreality. Or he may complain of indigestion, nausea, vomiting, abdominal cramps or diarrhoea. If the physician had good reason to initiate quinidine therapy in the first place he will often persist in the treatment in spite of the development of these symptoms. Quinidine may induce respiratory arrest in the experimental animal. There is reason to believe that it may have a similar effect in man. I recall one woman desperately ill with paroxysmal ventricular tachycardia in whom during the course of intravenous quinidine therapy respirations would stop, her head would turn to one side and her eyeballs roll upwards. On stopping the infusion respiration and other functions would return. Then on receiving the infusion at a slower drip rate she would do well for a time, then repeat the same sequence. Later a slower and persistently non-toxic rate was attained. Eventually she reverted to normal sinus rhythm. Most fatalities from intravenous quinidine occur in moribund patients. It seems quite possible that some of these fatalities are induced by respiratory arrest.

In the continental and South American literature there has been considerable interest in the use of intravenous magnesium sulfate (dose 2 to 4 grams as 20 or 50% solution), for ventricular tachycardia. This induces an unpleasant sense of suffusion and occasionally of nausea.[18] Though it has had a salutary effect on rare occasions, it has generally proven disappointing. This may be an unfair judgment for I have tended to use it as a last resort rather than early in the course of treatment. It may be recommended as a medication which one may try where others have failed.

In rare instances recalcitrant ventricular tachycardia has been treated by cervico-dorsal sympathectomy, generally unsuccessfully.

The paroxysmal ventricular tachycardia or ventricular flutter, which occurs as an advanced manifestation of potassium intoxication, should be treated by the measures outlined on page 160.

As indicated above (p. 207) it has recently been recommended that all patients with tachycardia who are hypotensive should first be treated with vaso-pressor amines before proceeding with the various antiarrhythmic agents already enumerated. Of all tachycardias it is in this group of paroxysmal ventricular tachycardia that shock is particularly prone to develop. My experience with this technique, though limited, seems to support this view.

In patients with paroxysmal ventricular tachycardia the existence of shock should, in the absence of another obvious or discernible cause, be attributed to the tachycardia itself and therapy should be directed accordingly. If the patient remains in shock after the subsidence of the tachycardia another cause of the shock, such as concealed hemorrhage or pulmonary or myocardial infarction, should be sought.

In ventricular tachycardia which has developed as a probable or certain consequence of digitalis overdosage or, in digitalized individuals who have somehow become depleted of potassium, digitalis should be omitted and potassium given in accordance with the recommendations given on p. 169. If potassium is ineffective quinidine or procaine amide may be used. In view of its almost invariable relationship to digitalis intoxication, these considerations are particularly pertinent in the case of alternating bidirectional tachycardia. It is also worth-while to try the effect of vagal maneuvers such as deep inspiration or carotid sinus stimulation in this ominous disturbance.

As indicated above there will inevitably be some cases in which the differentiation between paroxysmal ventricular tachycardia and supraventricular tachycardia with intraventricular block is impossible. In such cases, if the ventricular rhythm is slightly irregular, if there are slight variations in the intensity of the first sound and if the electrocardiogram shows bizarre ventricular complexes of varying form, it is justifiable to make the simpler deduction of paroxysmal ventricular tachycardia, and to treat it as such, than the more complex deduction which is based upon two assumptions, namely the existence of supraventricular tachycardia and intraventricular block. If the tachycardia persists despite all the measures enumerated above, and the patient is doing badly, it may then be justifiable to take the opposite gamble, assume supraventricular tachycardia and treat with digitalis.

REFERENCES

(1) Armbrust, C. A., Jr. and Levine, S. A.: Paroxysmal ventricular tachycardia: A study of one hundred and seven cases. Circ. 1: 28, 1950.

(2) Langendorf, R.: Auricular fibrillation with anomalous A-V conduction (WPW syndrome) imitating ventricular paroxysmal tachycardia. Am. Ht. J. 37: 645, 1949.

(3) Levine, S. A.: The clinical recognition of the various types of paroxysmal rapid heart action. Boston M. & S. J. 184: 53, 1921.

(4) Strong, G. F. and Levine, S. A.: The irregularity of the ventricular rate in paroxysmal ventricular tachycardia. Heart 10: 125, 1923.

(5) Levine, S. A.: The clinical recognition of paroxysmal ventricular tachycardia. Am. Ht. J. 3: 177, 1927.

(6) Gallavardin, L.: Tachycardie paroxystique ventriculaire. Arch. d. mal. du coeur. *13*: 121, 1920.

(7) Prinzmetal, M. and Kelley, F.: On the significance of the jugular pulse in the diagnosis of ventricular tachycardia. Am. Ht. J. *9*: 370, 1934.

(8) Katz, L. N. and Pick, A.: Clinical Electrocardiography. Part I. The Arrhythmias. Lea and Febiger, Philadelphia, 1956. p. 291.

(9) Ref. 8, p. 289.

(10) Scherf, D. and Kisch, F.: Ventricular tachycardia with variform ventricular complexes. Bull. N.Y. M. Coll., Flower and Fifth Ave. Hospitals *2*: 73, 1939.

(11) Zimdahl, W. T. and Kramer, L. I.: On the mechanism of paroxysmal tachycardia with rhythmic alternation in the direction of the ventricular complexes. Am. Ht. J. *33*: 218, 1947.

(12) Velasquez, J. and Kelser, G. A., Jr.: Alternating bidirectional tachycardia. Am. Ht. J. *54*: 440, 1957.

(13) Salley, S. M.: An unusual atropine effect on ventricular tachycardia. Am. J. Med. Sci. *183*: 456, 1932.

(14) Embree, L. J. and Levine, S. A.: Ventricular tachycardia: a case requiring massive amounts of procaine amide (Pronestyl) for reversion. Ann. Int. Med. *50*: 222, 1959.

(15) Schoolman, H., Pascale, L. R., Bernstein, L. M. and Littman, A.: Arterenol as an adjunct to the treatment of paroxysmal tachycardia. Am. Ht. J. *46*: 146, 1953.

(16) Kayden, H. J., Steele, J. M., Mark, L. C. and Brodie, B. B.: The use of procaine amide in cardiac arrhythmias. Circulation *4*: 13, 1951.

(17) Anderson, R. M., Boone, J. A. and Coleman, R. R.: The use of procaine amide in ventricular tachycardia. Southern Med. J. *44*: 905, 1951.

(18) Boyd, L. J. and Scherf, D.: Magnesium sulfate in paroxysmal tachycardia. Am. J. Med. Sci. *206*: 43, 1943.

[287]

(19) Davis, D. and Sprague, H. B.: Ventricular fibrillation: its relation to heart block. Am. Ht. J. 4: 559, 1929.

(20) Schwartz, S. P. and Jezer, A.: The action of quinine and quinidine on patients with transient ventricular fibrillation. Am. Ht. J. 9: 792, 1934.

(21) Corday, E., Gold, H., deVrea, L. B., Williams, J. H. and Fields, J.: Effect of the cardiac arrhythmias on the coronary circulation. Ann. Int. Med. 50: 539, 1959.

14

ADAMS - STOKES DISEASE

Diagnosis

Management

Ventricular Tachysystole in Complete Heart Block

14

ADAMS - STOKES DISEASE

The patient with atrioventricular heart block may develop standstill of the ventricles and unconsciousness through a number of different mechanisms. Starting with a normal sinus rhythm and delayed A-V conduction time (first degree A-V block), he may pass rapidly through a phase of second degree A-V block in which some of the atrial impulses do not get through to the ventricles, then to complete failure of the ventricles to respond to the auricular impulses (complete or third degree A-V block); at this time there may be a time-lag before the A-V node or a subsidiary ventricular pacemaker, at its inherently slow rate, assumes control of the ventricular rhythm. During this delay there is, for a time, no ventricular contraction and no cerebral blood flow. The suspended ventricular activity may be brief and occasion only a little dizziness or a "wave" and resemble a bout of petit mal. Or the pause may be protracted and associated with unconsciousness, cyanosis, convulsions or coma. If and when a new ventricular or nodal pacemaker resumes control of the ventricular rhythm at a fast enough rate, the patient recovers consciousness. If this does not occur after several minutes the patient dies. The whole process may repeat itself at shorter or longer intervals, giving rise to a succession of syncopal episodes. In this instance asystole occurs during the transition from partial to complete heart block.

Complete heart block may, alternatively, be of long standing and the usual ventricular rate fast enough, say, 32 to 35 beats per minute, to sustain an adequate peripheral and central circulation. If now the nodal or ventricular pacemaker suddenly fails to generate an impulse and, at the same time, no other subsidiary ventricular pacemaker "escapes," a similar standstill of the ventricles develops. Again if the vital brain centers are deprived of an adequate supply of oxygen for more than a few seconds, the patient loses consciousness. Ordinarily this comes on without warning and the patient may injure himself.

On rare occasions the rhythm may change in the space of one beat directly from a sinus mechanism without A-V delay to complete standstill of the ventricles (Fig. 36,B); on recovery a normal sinus mechanism may immediately be re-established. In such a case the physician who arrives at the scene moments after the patient's recovery will be unable, even with the benefit of an electrocardiogram, to establish the mechanism of the patient's attack. A clue that the syncopal attack was due to complete heart block may be the development of complete heart block on carotid sinus stimulation;[1] this response is not elicited in the normal heart. At times the syncopal attack is due, not to standstill, but to excessive slowing of the ventricles. The result is the same, inadequate cerebral blood flow. Recovery does not follow until the old or a new pacemaker discharges at a rate sufficient to maintain an adequate output. Palpitation may be the presenting symptom, or an important symptom, in complete heart block. Even before he has formed the habit of counting his radial pulse rate, the patient has long been aware of the slowing of his heart in his breast.

In many cases of established complete heart block syncope is due neither to excessive slowing nor to actual standstill of the ventricles, but to the opposite extreme, namely an excessively rapid heart rate. This may be the result of transient ventricular tachycardia (Figs. 37 and 38) or flutter or even of

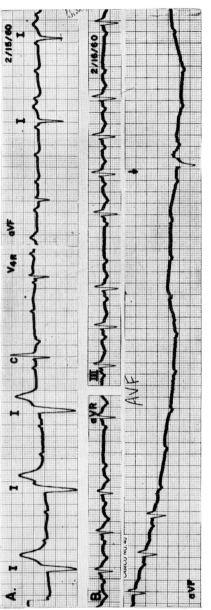

Fig. 36. Syncopal attacks during recession of complete heart block in a 64-year-old man with coronary artery disease and Adams-Stokes attacks of several months' duration. Sodium lactate, chlorothiazide and cortisone without demonstrable effect on rate or paroxysms. Latter controlled with Isuprel. (A) Tracings, recorded when patient free of attacks for one week, show transitions between complete A-V block (ventricular rate 45) and second degree (partial) A-V block. QRS during complete block shows configuration of left bundle branch block (I), while conducted beats (C) show configuration of right bundle branch block. (B) Tracings on following day show second degree A-V block and right bundle branch block. The P-R interval of conducted beats is 0.16 second. The lower strip shows the abrupt transition from normal A-V conduction to complete ventricular standstill. The single ventricular escape beat recorded in this strip resulted from a blow to the chest (arrow). A few beats later spontaneous resumption of normal sinus rhythm immediately with normal P-R interval. If electrocardiogram were recorded only before or after syncopal attack, complete block might not have been suspected.

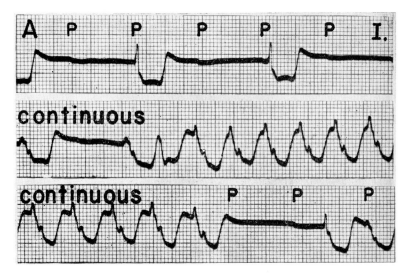

Fig. 37 *Paroxysmal ventricular tachycardia developing on a background of complete heart block* in patient with acute posterior myocardial infarction (Continuous strips) Ventricular rate during complete block 42, during ventricular tachycardia 160. These paroxysms appeared to be controlled by rations of epinephrine

[294]

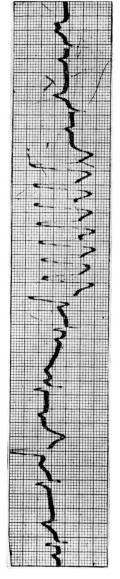

Fig. 38. Short *paroxysm of ventricular tachycardia in patient with underlying complete A-V block* Ventricular premature beats preceding and following such paroxysms show a configuration identical with the QRS complexes of the paroxysm and may be regarded as a clue, not completely reliable, that the syncopal attacks were due not to standstill but to ventricular tachysystole. Patient at times aware of tachycardia. The salvo was associated with dizziness; longer attacks not illustrated were accompanied by syncope. They seemed to be controlled with epinephrine but the patient died later of ventricular fibrillation.

transient ventricular fibrillation. It has been said that these mechanisms explain about half of the syncopal attacks occurring in complete heart block [2] but in my experience such mechanisms have been much less frequent than standstill or slowing of the heart. Some patients may lose consciousness during the tachycardia, others only during the period of standstill which follows so frequently after the tachycardia.

Complete heart block is most commonly the result of coronary artery disease. It may develop during an acute episode of myocardial infarction, particularly that variety affecting the posterior wall. (Fig. 37.) This is a serious complication and carries a grave prognosis. But if the patient recovers from the acute attack the complete block disappears. This condition is somewhat more common in patients with chronic coronary artery disease and myocardial fibrosis who do not remember ever having suffered an acute heart attack. It can also occur in hypertensive or rheumatic valvular heart disease but is extremely rare during active rheumatic carditis. It is occasionally observed in patients who have had diphtheria and, very rarely, after syphilis. An oft-cited gumma of the upper part of the interventricular septum, presumably interrupting the A-V bundle, is illustrated in a textbook on physical diagnosis in common use a generation ago.[3] There is some suggestive evidence [4] that Adams-Stokes attacks may be triggered by the presence of stones in the gall-bladder and that these attacks may be prevented by cholecystectomy. Complete heart block is seen only rarely as a consequence of digitalis intoxication. When it does occur under these circumstances it does not generally induce syncope, perhaps because of the tendency of patients in this digitalis group to have a faster ventricular rate even though they are in complete block. Patients with congenital complete heart block likewise have a relatively rapid ventricular rate and little tendency to syncope.[5]

[296]

DIAGNOSIS

The recognition of complete atrioventricular block goes a long way toward determining the background, if not the immediate mechanism, of syncope. The atria are activated from the sino-atrial node at a normal rate, generally somewhere between 70 and 90. At the same time the ventricles are driven by a nodal or ventricular pacemaker, commonly at a rate below 50. The ventricular rate is accelerated very little, if at all, by such influences as exercise, fever, atropine or epinephrine, which speed up the normal ventricle. The atria may be regular or show sinus arrhythmia; the ventricles may be perfectly regular, or show a minor and subtle irregularity. In the electrocardiogram the atrial deflections (P waves) and the ventricular deflections (QRS complexes) are quite independent of each other. The ventricular complexes may be identical with those of conducted beats shown in the same lead at other times (nodal beats) or they may be abnormal in appearance resembling those of right or left bundle branch block ("idioventricular beats"). These are inscribed at a slow rate and, with the qualification stated above, at a regular rhythm. The rate of the atria is faster than that of the ventricles. The QRS complexes being quite independent of the P waves, the latter bear a random relationship to the QRS complexes, sometimes preceding, sometimes following and sometimes coinciding with, but generally not influencing them.

The independence of the atrial and ventricular rhythms explains some of the bedside features of this disturbance. Because the atria and ventricles beat independently of one another there is a varying time relationship between atrial and ventricular contraction. We have seen (p. 222) that the intensity of the first heart sound is dependent upon atrioventricular conduction time. When the P-R interval is short, say 0.12 or 0.14 second, the sound is accentuated; when longer, say 0.19 or 0.24 second, it is decreased in intensity. Consequently there is considerable variation in the loudness of the first sound in complete block. In fact with some of the shorter P-R intervals S_1 may become tremendously accentuated and booming in quality and aptly described as a "bruit de canon". If the atria are fibrillating such changes in the intensity of S_1 cannot be detected. Another auscultatory feature, likewise conditioned by the independence of the atrial and ventricular rhythm, is the presence of atrial sounds during ventricular diastole. Their detection frequently requires the utmost of attention but at times they are so loud as to be mistaken for premature ventricular beats, especially since the atrial contractions occurring early in diastole are generally heard much more readily than those occurring late in diastole. Frequently it is possible in complete block to observe "a" waves in the neck veins; the impulses are faster than the apex beat, simultaneously seen, felt or heard, and have a rhythm independent of the apex rate.

During the attack of syncope one may note pronounced ventricular slowing or silence of the ventricles; in rare cases one may hear the tattoo of ventricular tachycardia. But frequently respirations are so noisy that it is impossible to be sure just what the heart is doing. In any case, it is always desirable if not mandatory to record an electrocardiogram during an attack or after.

MANAGEMENT

It is the emergency management of the syncopal attack itself which principally concerns us here. It is important, first of all, to take all necessary measures to prevent injury to the patient. This means that side-rails will be kept in position when the patient is unattended. One then asks which of the two possible types of mechanism described above is responsible for the attack. For the patient with recurrent bouts of standstill or of excessive slowing, pharmacologic or electrophysical measures are available. These may be given in tandem or together. The availability of the necessary apparatus, the experience of the physician and the efficacy of previous therapy will largely govern treatment.

In the pharmaco-therapeutic category are included those drugs which are capable of awakening normal nodal or idioventricular pacemakers, or, if these are already active but sluggish, of speeding up their rate. In patients with frequent episodes of ventricular standstill epinephrine (1:1000) or isopropyl-arterenol (Isuprel) (1:5000), (0.3 to 0.5 cc. of either) may be injected subcutaneously at intervals adequate to prevent excessive slowing or standstill. Just how often this must be done, and in what dose, must be determined by trial and error. If the patient does well for, say, three hours, then three and a half hours after his last dose begins afresh to have seizures, the appropriate interval would be three hours between injections. The interval, be it noted, may vary from time to time. Occasionally it will be necessary to repeat the dose as frequently as every hour. Ectopic ventricular beats may be an unpleasant side effect during this titration; the dose should be cut down in the event of their development. This technique of repeated subcutaneous injection must subject the heart to a waxing and waning concentration of the drug. This may be evened out, in part at least, by the intramuscular injection of adrenalin in oil (1 cc. contains 2 mgms.) once or twice a day. Better still, the heart may be subjected to a relatively unchanging concentration of the drug if it is given in an intravenous infusion. To this end one may add 4 cc. of 1:1000 epinephrine to one liter of 5% dextrose in water and run the solution in by vein, starting the infusion at a rate of 15 drops a minute, increasing the rate of infusion according to the response of the heart rate and aiming at a rate of 35 to 40 beats per minute. The infusion is stopped temporarily in the event of ectopic activity, excessive rise in blood pressure or excessive cerebral stimulation, and resumed at a slower rate on their disappearance. When the heart rate has become stable an attempt is made to cut down on the rate of flow and eventually, after hours or days, the patient is weaned from this treatment altogether.

As an alternative to epinephrine one may use isopropyl arterenol (Isuprel). This is preferred in hypertensive patients since, unlike epinephrine, it has no vaso-pressor action.[6] On the other hand, epinephrine will be preferred over isopropylarterenol in complete heart block complicating acute myocardial infarction or complicated by shock for the very reason that is is a superior vaso-pressor agent. Isuprel is available in ampoules of 0.2 mgm. each. One dissolves the contents of five such ampoules in 250 cc. of dextrose in water and governs the rate of flow as indicated above under epinephrine. Much of the literature to the contrary notwithstanding, Isuprel has a less pronounced but still definite propensity to induce ectopic rhythms.

In those cases where the syncopal seizures occur as a result of asystole during the transition from partial to complete A-V block full digitalization given during complete block may render the complete block persistent and permanent and the clinical state of the patient more stable and less vulnerable to periods of standstill.[7] There is some difference of opinion about whether digitalis should be used at all in patients with complete heart block. I have seen no harm and much good done when this drug is used for congestive heart failure complicating or complicated by complete block. In my experience, even when it brings about no significant changes in the heart rate digitalis can increase the cardiac output under these circumstances.

Where the sympathico-mimetic amines fail to accelerate or rouse the ventricles or where toxic symptoms develop along with effective therapeutic response, recourse may be had to the external stimulator or "pacemaker".[8] This should be available in running condition and located as close to all hospital wards and rooms as feasible. Since this is generally impractical it is wise to have more than one at hand. All medical and surgical internes should be taught the technique of resuscitation, including the use of the pacemaker, early in their careers. The method of using the pacemaker should be redemonstrated periodically to the house staff. One electrode is applied with electrode paste to the region of the cardiac apex and the other similarly to a corresponding region over the right chest. These electrodes should be held in place by rubber straps which encircle the patient's chest. (Fig. 39.) An electrocardiogram should also be attached, recording one lead, generally Lead aVF at half normal standardization. AC interference is avoided by connecting the electrocardiograph to the "pacemaker" with a wire and grounding the "pacemaker" to an external ground. The patient in turn is grounded by the negative output wire from the pacemaker. The pacemaker is turned on to 60 cycles per minute and the amplitude, starting from zero, is progressively increased with each impulse until a premature beat is induced by the external stimulus. The strength of stimulation is maintained just above the threshold thus determined. If the heart is already beating spontaneously at a slow rate there may, for a time, be a competition between the spontaneous and the induced beats. The introduced beats which fall in the refractory period of the spontaneous beats will be ineffective. But those falling in the responsive phase are generally followed by a response. Since electrical response does not always signify a mechanical response, it is desirable to check whether the induced beat recorded electrocardiographically is associated with a blood pressure response. The stimulus induces contraction of skeletal as well as cardiac muscle. It thus produces a jerk of the chest wall muscles which may be painful. This may be minimized by the use of chloral hydrate or Dem-

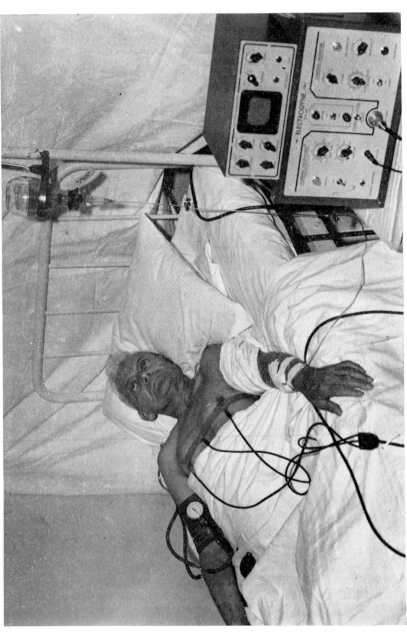

Fig. 39. Patient with recurrent Adams-Stokes attacks with "pacemaker" recording action potential on lag screen. Single heart beats signalled by flashing light and beeping sound mechanism. Infusion of Isuprel running into vein on left forearm. Blood pressure cuff in place on opposite arm. Since attendant is present side-rails are down.

erol. As he becomes accustomed to it the patient generally complains less of this symptom. In a rare case these violent muscular contractions make it necessary to abandon the use of the "pacemaker."

An attempt is made to keep the rate of stimulation between 35 and 45. Stimulation is discontinued periodically and tentatively to observe whether spontaneous beats are resumed. If these do not appear after 2 or 3 seconds the pacemaker is started again. In the meantime one of the sympathico-mimetic amines may be given as described above to nudge ventricular pacemakers.

Once the immediate emergency of recurrent or persistent standstill or slowing has been met it is wise to continue with the milder sympathico-mimetic amines for long-term therapy. Capsules of ephedrine sulfate (25 to 50 mgms.) by mouth, sublingual tablets (Glossets) of Isuprel (10–15 mgms.) dissolved under the tongue or in the cheek pouch or swallowed, or inhalations of 1:100 epinephrine, may be tried every four hours or so. But there would seem to be little justification for their use when attacks are frequent or prolonged. Atropine in therapeutic dosage (1 to 2 mgms.) or as tincture of belladonna in tolerated and effective dosage, may be given alone or in combination with the sympathico-mimetic amines, but these agents are only very rarely effective. Their use is more justifiable if in the past the patient has shown spontaneous lapses into lesser degrees of block or if a changing degree of block has been demonstrated on deliberate carotid sinus stimulation. One must bear in mind the wakefulness or urinary retention which may be induced by the pressor amines and the dryness and photophobia which may follow the use of atropine and related substances.

Bellet and his co-workers [9] have reported an encouraging experience with molar sodium lactate in arousing or accelerating ventricular pacemakers. The recommended dose is 70 to 200 cc.

[303]

given by vein at a rate of 7 to 30 cc. per minute. With one exception my experience with this substance has been disappointing. I must confess that in most of the patients in whom I have tried sodium lactate other forms of therapy have already been tried, likewise ineffectually. Nevertheless it may be worth-while keeping this compound in mind.

Cortisone is capable of shortening the P-R interval of the normal individual [10] and of the patient with Addison's disease.[11] It may be conjectured that this could be a more universal property of the steroids, perhaps making them effective in high grades of atrioventricular block. A limited personal experience with this substance in complete heart block has been disappointing. It is possible that the reported efficacy of ACTH in Adams-Stokes attacks of infective or rheumatic origin [12] is related to suppression of infection rather than to the above described effect upon atrioventricular conduction.

VENTRICULAR TACHYSYSTOLE IN COMPLETE HEART BLOCK

Appropriate therapy is ill-defined and controversial when the syncopal attacks are due to paroxysmal ventricular tachycardia or paroxysmal ventricular fibrillation developing in a background of complete heart block. There are reasonable theoretical [13] and valid practical [14,15] objections to the use of quinidine or procaine amide in this emergency. These agents depress the junctional tissues as well as the myocardium proper. And in the presence of complete atrioventricular block or of intraventricular block experience indicates that they may somehow precipitate ventricular tachycardia, fibrillation or standstill. On the other hand it is generally held that epinephrine has a definite tendency to excite lower ventricular pacemakers even when an idioventricular pacemaker is already established. Faced with this dilemma some authorities prefer to do nothing.

It is known that in normal sinus rhythm ventricular premature beats are prone to emerge when the heart rate is slow, to disappear as the heart speeds up. By analogy if pressor amines can rouse a nodal pacemaker during complete block, it is conceivable that the tendency to complicating ventricular ectopic rhythms could be suppressed [7,16] by these drugs. There is some evidence that isopropylarterenol can stimulate active ventricular pacemakers without exciting lower ventricular foci.[16] To the extent that this is valid (and my experience suggests that this is not invariably true) the use of Isuprel has been recommended in this situation. I have seen two patients in whom this form of therapy seemed to be effective. The period of asystole which follows ventricular tachycardia is generally brief and self-limited. If this exceeds a few seconds the chest should be struck a smart blow (Fig. 40), or the heart stimulated with a needle or the external pacemaker, already attached and ready for operation, should be used. If this is not at hand, epinephrine or one of the other sympathicomimetic drugs described above should be injected intracardially. One hesitates to recommend thoracotomy on the ward at this juncture for fear of abuse of the procedure; this subject is discussed at length on page 347. In desperate cases the external defibrillator may be used to terminate ventricular tachycardia or fibrillation complicating complete block.[17] The technique of its use is described on page 347. When the ventricles have become quiescent the external pacemaker is promptly used to initiate cardiac contraction and restore a normal cardiac mechanism.

When it is not known whether the attacks are due to slowing or standstill on the one hand, or to ventricular tachycardia or fibrillation on the other, it seems a reasonable gamble to consider the detection of ventricular premature beats a clue that tachycardia or fibrillation is responsible for the syncope. If ventricular premature beats are not heard and the mecha-

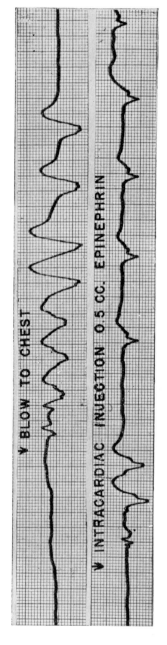

Fig. 40. *Emergency Therapy in Cardiac Standstill.* The patient was a 67 year old man with old and fresh myocardial infarction who developed repetitive syncope. No heart block. Upper tracing shows "paradoxical" effect of blow to chest in converting standstill to slow fibrillation of the ventricles. The risk of such response should be accepted (Scherf). The lower strip recorded immediately thereafter shows resumption of slow idio-ventricular rhythm after intracardiac injection of 0.5 cc. of epinephrine (1:1000).

nisms of the syncopal attacks has not been determined, it would seem a reasonable guess that they result from standstill. In all honesty, however, it must be stated that some patients show one mechanism at one time, and the opposite mechanism at another time, even moments later, and therefore that electro-cardiographic monitoring is most desirable. Isuprel would appear to be the therapy of choice under two circumstances: (1) where it is not known whether the attacks are due to slowing or standstill or to ventricular tachycardia or fibrillation: or (2) where it is known that the patient actually exhibits slow mechanisms in some of the attacks and fast mechanisms in others.

So unpredictable is the return of attacks that it is difficult if not impossible to know when the emergency has ceased. For months the sword of Damocles hangs over the patient's head. The disheartening experience of having the patient succumb on the eve of departure from the hospital or shortly after his arrival home is not rare. Though one may have some qualms about its effect upon the patient's morale, it seems wise to have "pacemaker" and epinephrine constantly at hand until the patient has had no attack for two weeks. Even then ambulation will be undertaken with trepidation. As a possible aid for some of these patients an extremely intriguing research is in progress. This concerns the feasibility of embedding in the heart an electrode which can, directly or by induction, be stimulated by a portable battery. In the event of real or imminent syncope the patient or an attendant could stimulate the heart to beat at an optimal rate. Certain technical difficulties have yet to be ironed out to make this persistently effective but there have already been a number of favorable reports on the use of such a device.

There is, of course, a limit beyond which one cannot go. The decision will eventually have to be taken to have the patient do without his walker, nurse, attendant or "pace-

maker." The most cheering aspect of these cases is that somehow the survivors of these attacks do well after the lapse of
months even though they continue to exhibit heart block.

REFERENCES

(1) Penton, G. B., Miller, H. and Levine, S. A.: Some clinical
features of complete heart block. Circulation, *13*: 801,
1956.

(2) Parkinson, J., Papp, C. and Evans, W.: The electrocardiogram of the Stokes-Adams attack. Brit. Ht. J. *3*: 171, 1941.

(3) Norris, G. W. and Landis, H. R. M.: Diseases of the
Chest and the Principles of Physical Diagnosis. W. B.
Saunders, Philadelphia and London. (Fourth Edition)
1929, p. 776.

(4) McLemore, G. A. and Levine, S. A.: The possible therapeutic value of cholecystectomy in Adams-Stokes disease.
Am. J. Med. Sci. 229: 386, 1955.

(5) Levine, H. D.: A case of congenital complete heart block
with labile ventricular rate. Am. Ht. J. *10*: 376, 1935.

(6) Zoll, P. M., Linenthal, A. J., Gibson, W., Paul, M. H. and
Norman, L. R.: Intravenous drug therapy of Stokes-
Adams disease. Effects of sympathomimetic amines on
ventricular rhythmicity and atrioventricular conduction.
Circulation, *17*: 325, 1958.

(7) Wright, J. C., Hejtmoncik, M. D., Herrmann, G. R. and
Shields, A. H.: A clinical study of complete heart block.
Am. Ht. J. *52*: 369, 1956.

(8) Zoll, P. M., Linenthal, A. J. and Norman, L. R.: Treatment of Stokes-Adams disease by external electric stimulation of the heart. Circulation, 9: 482, 1954.

(9) Bellet, S., Wasserman, F. and Brody, J. I.: Treatment of
cardiac arrest and slow ventricular rates in complete

heart block. Use of molar and half-molar sodium lactate; a clinical study. Circulation, *11*: 685, 1955.

(10) Lown, B., Arons, W. L., Ganong, W. F., Vazifdar, J. P. and Levine, S. A.: Adrenal steroids and auriculoventricular conduction. Am. Ht. J. *50*: 760, 1955.

(11) Somerville, W., Levine, H. D. and Thorn, G. W.: The electrocardiogram in Addison's Disease. Medicine *30*: 43, 1951.

(12) Litchfield, J. W., Manley, K. A. and Polak, A.: Stokes-Adams attacks treated with corticotrophin. Lancet, *1*: 935, 1958.

(13) Davis, D. and Sprague, H. B.: Ventricular fibrillation: its relation to heart block. Am. Ht. J. *4*: 559, 1929.

(14) Schwartz, S. P., Hallinger, L. and Imperialli, A.: Transient ventricular fibrillation. IV. The effects of procaine amide on patients with transient ventricular fibrillation during established auriculo-ventricular dissociation. Circulation, *6*: 193, 1952.

(15) Schwartz, S. P. and Jezer, A.: The action of quinine and quinidine on patients with transient ventricular fibrillation. Am. Ht. J. *9*: 792, 1934.

(16) Robbin, S. R., Goldfine, S., Schwartz, M. J. and Dack, S.: Adams-Stokes syndrome. The treatment of ventricular asystole, ventricular tachycardia and ventricular fibrillation associated with complete heart block. Am. J. Med. *18*: 577, 1955.

(17) Zoll, P. M., Linenthal, A., Zarsky, L. R. N.: Ventricular fibrillation: treatment and prevention by external electric currents. N.E.J. Med. *262*: 105, 1960.

Vaso-Depressor Syncope

Syncope due to Impaired Venous Return

Cardiac Syncope

Cerebral Syncope

15

SYNCOPE

Syncope is here regarded as an abruptly developing, complete and transient loss of consciousness. If the period of unconsciousness lasts long enough, convulsions may follow. The fact should be emphasized that convulsions may occur in syncope of any cause and do not necessarily indicate disease of the central nervous system. In certain conditions syncope develops when the subject has exerted himself beyond a certain point. Stopping short of this threshold may prevent the faint; exceeding it may bring on the faint. Under certain circumstances syncope may be related to the posture of the patient, developing more certainly, readily or promptly in the upright than in the recumbent position.

The ultimate mechanism of syncope is a disturbance in the nutrition or blood supply to vital brain centers. This may come about through a number of mechanisms. Physiologists have conceded that in some forms of syncope the mechanism is obscure or complicated. Classifications have therefore been attempted on the basis of what is regarded as the fundamental or underlying mechanism. For the sake of convenience in presentation such a tentative scheme is followed here. In general syncope may be regarded as developing as the result of a fall in the systemic blood pressure level as a result of a disturbance in one of three principal functions: (1) *by producing*

[313]

peripheral vascular collapse (vaso-depressor syncope, anaphylactic shock); (2) *by a decrease in the venous return to the heart*. This acts by diminishing left ventricular filling, cardiac output, aortic flow and thus cerebral perfusion; and (3) *by inducing primary impairment of cardiac output* ("Cardiac syncope"). This refers to changes in the cardiac output and cerebral blood flow dependent upon structural or functional abnormalities resident in the heart itself. The final common path in these three mechanisms is a drop in systemic blood pressure. There is a fourth group in which syncope occurs as a consequence of abnormal intracranial or cerebral processes.

VASO-DEPRESSOR SYNCOPE

The *simple faint* (benign syncope, psychogenic syncope), such as that occurring at the sight of blood or during or after a venipuncture is probably due to vagal inhibition. In subjects with this disturbance Sir Thomas Lewis [1] demonstrated simultaneous vasodilatation and vagal bradycardia and therefore designated it as the vaso-vagal syndrome. If timely observations are possible, a sharp bradycardia is demonstrated to precede the depressor response. Initially the blood pressure level is defended, then there is a marked depressor response due apparently to acute vasodilatation into muscle vessels.[2] Fainting, of course, places the patient in a horizontal position. This, of itself, restores adequate cerebral circulation. Hence a "built-in" feature of the attack is its own treatment. Following such an attack it is probably wise to avoid the circumstances that led to the attack, to keep the patient seated for a time with his head between his knees or even to have him lie down for a while.

Carotid sinus syncope is said to come about in part as a result of reflexly induced bradycardia or asystole [3,4] but this may be associated with the same sort of vaso-depressor reflex as that just described. In the experimental preparation, stimulation of the aortic baro-receptors,[5] particularly those of the carotid sinus, can induce two types of response, namely a fall in blood pressure and cardiac slowing or standstill. These two effects may be combined in the same subject. There is said to be a third type of carotid sinus syncope associated with neither hypotension nor bradycardia and presumably due to some direct impairment in cerebral blood flow; there is very little convincing evidence that such a condition exists. In many alleged instances such syncope may be caused by throttling of cerebral blood flow by manual compression of the carotid artery, particularly if the blood supply to the opposite side of the brain is already compromised. When carotid sinus sensitivity is suspected, an attempt should be made to demonstrate its presence by deliberate stimulation of the carotid sinus. But it must be emphasized that this is not without some hazard; in rare instances it has induced cerebral thrombosis or even a fatality. A practical method for detecting carotid sinus sensitivity is for the observer to listen to the apex rate while he stimulates the carotid sinus. If the heart slows appreciably or goes into standstill and, at the same time, the patient develops such symptoms as giddiness, dizziness, lightheadedness or faintness, similar to, or identical with, the symptoms of which he has complained, he probably has a sensitive carotid sinus. If he should develop such symptoms without appreciable slowing of the heart, the procedure should be repeated while observations are made of the blood pressure. It is important to bear in mind, as pointed out above, that the blood pressure may fall merely and secondarily as a result of the cardiac slowing. I know of no reliable criteria [6] related to the degree of slowing or fall in blood pressure which establish that an individual does or does not have a sensitive carotid sinus. This must be a subjective evaluation. A "full dress" test for carotid sinus sensitivity may be made simultaneously by three observers, one stimulating the carotid sinus while his stethoscope is held to the precordium, the second recording the blood pressure and the third counting the apical heart rate or recording a continuous electrocardiogram. The patient is seated upright in bed in such a position that he will not be hurt should he fall. After a baseline heart rate and blood pressure have been determined the first observer massages the carotid sinus (see page 204) in a rotatory manner for no longer than five seconds. The blood pressure and the heart rate (or electrocardiogram) are recorded during and after that period. It may be necessary to stimulate sequentially at more than one site on one side, or on the opposite side before an abnormal response is elicited. Carotid sinus sensitivity is extremely difficult if not impossible to standardize. Many alleged instances of changing carotid sinus sensitivity, even when observed by the same individual, are the result of varying site, intensity, manner or briskness of stimulation. Furthermore the mere demonstration of carotid sinus sensitivity in a given patient does not establish that this is necessarily the cause of his syncopal attacks. In many people this mechanism, though demonstrable, has not produced symptoms. Even the induction of symptoms identical with the presenting complaint does not prove that they are necessarily due to carotid sinus sensitivity. But this inference will seem more logical. Demonstrable carotid sinus sensitivity may persist though the patient, either spontaneously or as a result of treatment, no longer has syncopal attacks. Alternatively he may, with the passage of time, lose his sensitivity. In my experience a considerable proportion of patients with carotid sinus sensitivity have, in addition to this condition, functional hypoglycemia.

Treatment consists of the oral administration of atropine (0.5 to 0.75 mgm.) or of tincture of belladonna (increasing from 10 to 45 drops t.i.d. as tolerated and until effective) and ephedrine 25 to 50 mgm. 4 i.d.; these measures are combined with a high-protein diet. The latter minimizes any tendency to

functional hypoglycemia. Although in earlier experiences denervation of the carotid sinus and, more recently, irradia-
tion of the sinus or intracranial section of the glosso-pharyngeal
nerve,[7] have been performed, it has been my experience that
such drastic measures are rarely if ever necessary. At times the
surgical removal of a cervical tumor which impinges upon the
carotid sinus, or simply changing from a stiff to a soft collar, is
all that is necessary. A number of years ago I was called to see
a visitor who had fainted at a wedding dinner. He was wearing
an outgrown tuxedo with stiff collar and shirt, dating back,
perhaps, to his college years. The change to a soft shirt and correct collar size enabled him to continue without further
incident.

Hyperventilation Syncope

This infrequent cause of syncope is probably active through
the alkalosis resulting from blowing off excessive amounts of
carbon dioxide (hypocapnia).[8] The blood pressure always falls
in the faints due to hyperventilation; there is a dilatation of the
vascular bed in the muscles and, at the same time, cerebral
vasoconstriction. The presence of certain associated symptoms
often serves to alert the physician to the possibility that
reported or observed syncope is actually the result of hyperventilation. This includes faintness, dizziness, unsteadiness, numbness, tingling and coldness of hands, feet or face, particularly
in the perioral regions, muscular spasms, tremors, twitching,
rarely carpo-pedal spasm with generalized tetany, yawning,
a peculiar type of dyspnea described as a sensation of a need
to but an inability to draw a satisfactory breath, palpitation,
atypical chest pains, dryness of the mouth, dysphagia or
bloating. If a spontaneous attack is not observed the patient is
asked to overbreathe for three minutes. He may then develop
symptoms which he may admit, spontaneously or on question-

ing, are identical with those preceding some of his syncopal attacks. He is then asked to rebreathe from a paper bag. This is followed by prompt relief of symptoms. "To the patient the acute precipitation of his attack is both alarming and impressive, and its immediate termination with the paper bag technique is proportionately reassuring," [9] but this demonstration is rarely effective in curing the tendency to hyperventilation. Psychotherapy may be necessary. At times hyperventilation is related to salicylate ingestion.

Orthostatic hypotension The normal blood pressure response to the change from a reclining to a standing position is a slightly lowered systolic blood pressure and a slight elevation of the diastolic blood pressure. At times when this response is impaired, a fall of the systolic and diastolic blood pressure levels ensues. A slight fall may induce a little dizziness but patients whose pressure plummets toward or to zero may lose consciousness. There is generally a paltry rise in the heart rate despite the profound fall in blood pressure. This reaction results in the pooling of large amounts of blood in the lower parts of the body. Orthostatic hypotension is ordinarily the result of disorder in the autonomic nervous system from organic disease such as tabes dorsalis, multiple sclerosis, syringomyelia or diabetic neuropathy.[10] It is an expected phenomenon following thoraco-lumbar sympathectomy but I have recently seen a patient who first developed severe orthostatic hypotension with syncope after a bilateral lumbar sympathectomy for arteriosclerosis obliterans. Certain drugs such as morphine and other opiates, nitroglycerin (see page 55), quinidine, emetine and the hypotensive agents including the rauwolfia derivatives, the ganglionic blocking agents (apresoline) chlorothiazide and the tranquilizing agents, particularly chlorpromazine, have been known to produce orthostatic hypotension. This condition is also quite common as a temporary finding following severe illnesses requiring a long period of rest in bed. It is quite common as a transient phenomenon in "brittle" elderly patients in whom it may be related to peripheral arteriosclerosis and an "end organ" failure (vascular unresponsiveness). There are some individuals in whom orthostatic hypotension is combined with anhydrosis and sexual impotence; the cause of the hypotension is not clear in this group of patients. The detection of orthostatic hypotension should always lead to a thorough investigation for pheochromocytoma [11] or unilateral kidney disease.

If it is suspected that the reaction is due to any one of the drugs listed above, the drug or its dosage should be changed. These patients should be warned to avoid sudden changes in position and rather to climb from the reclining to the sitting and then to the standing position in slow easy stages. They may be helped by the wearing of an elastic girdle and elastic stockings extending from feet to mid-thigh. A pressurized "anti-gravity" suit, similar to that used in experimental space projects, has been suggested.[12] In addition atropine or belladonna and the pressor amines, notably ephedrine, are worthy of trial but are generally ineffective. "Salting up" the patient by liberalizing his intake of sodium chloride or by the prescription of salt-retaining steroids such as desoxycorticosterone in titrated dosage [13] or 9-alpha fluorohydrocortisone, 2.0 mgms. per day, gradually tapering to 0.1 mgm. daily,[14] may be tried. In the absence of a contraindication these patients should be maintained on an intake of 10 grams of salt a day when symptom-free. In some patients, notably the post-operative, post-infectious and the elderly group, the condition is a self-limited one, which improves regardless of therapy.

SYNCOPE DUE TO IMPAIRED VENOUS RETURN

The initiating event here is a critical fall in central venous pressure and consequent inadequate return of blood to the left ventricle, but this mechanism produces syncope through the same final common path as other conditions, namely a fall in the systemic blood pressure. This may be due to causes "proximal" to the right or left ventricle.

Oligemic Syncope This disturbance results from a loss of the effective blood volume. This may be due to an absolute blood loss as in hemorrhage,[15] or to a relative blood loss resulting from redistribution of blood. Slow chronic blood loss does not ordinarily induce syncope; the blood loss must be rapid. In all cases of unexplained syncope particular thought must be directed to the possibility of massive concealed internal hemorrhage. Treatment consists in control of the bleeding, whatever its source, and restoration of an adequate blood volume.

In other instances, though the total blood volume is normal, the effective blood volume may be diminished because of sequestration of blood in muscles or elsewhere. With extensive varicose veins the erect posture may pool an additional 500 to 900 cc. of blood in the legs,[16] with a corresponding decrease in the venous return to the heart. Such pooling is minimized by the use of elastic stockings or by appropriate surgery.

Though Hollywood still labors in the misbelief that syncope is a common feature of early pregnancy there is one form of syncope which does occur near term. This develops when the patient lies flat on her back. It is probably related, in large part at least, to the pressure of the gravid uterus upon the large pelvic veins and the consequent reduction in venous return. This can be avoided by advising the patient to lie on her side. Syncope from relative oligemia may also occur in shock, whether traumatic or "medical" or allergic. A special instance

of the latter is the syncope which may develop in cold urticaria involving large areas of the body surface.[17] A generalized
vascular collapse, due presumably to flooding with histamine
or histamine-like substances, may explain some of the drowning or near-drowning accidents which occur each year even
in excellent swimmers.[18]

Tussive Syncope This almost always affects extroverted,
middle-aged, slightly overweight and muscular men given to
excessive smoking and drinking and subject to pulmonary emphysema, bronchial asthma or frequent infections of the respiratory tract.[19] Thus physique, personality and respiratory pattern
alert the physician to the correct diagnosis. A scratchy sensation
in the throat often initiates the attack which generally consists
of a staccato series of dry coughs accompanied by violent muscular efforts. After a brief or prolonged salvo the coughing
paroxysm ceases, the patient stops breathing, becomes slightly
dizzy and the vision dims. He may then lose consciousness. If
standing, he falls, if sitting he slumps, or, when reclining, the
head falls back. The face becomes suffused at first, later pale,
and sweating ensues. In a small percentage of cases convulsions
have been described. The attack generally lasts no longer than
a few seconds, the patient revives quite unaware of having
"blacked out" and resumes his previous activity. In a few cases
injuries have been sustained.

Cough apparently has two important effects upon the cardiovascular system. During the coughing paroxysm marked elevation may develop in the intrapleural, arterial pulmonary and
right ventricular pressure. (Valsalva maneuver). The extremely
high intrathoracic pressure obstructs venous return at the
thoracic inlet.[20,2] This is probably the more important
mechanism. The second effect is a profound fall in the systemic
blood pressure. This may be precipitated reflexly through the
large increase in carotid sinus pressure that may be induced
by the cough itself. There is some experimental evidence also

that the pulmonary vessels may be the site of receptors which, when stimulated by a rise in the mean pressure in the pulmonary circuit, initiate strong cardiovascular reflexes [5] and peripheral vaso-dilatation. The possible rôle of such reflexes in tussive syncope remains to be elucidated. There is finally some evidence that tremendous increases in both arterial blood pressure and in jugular pressure during the act of coughing may effectively and directly throttle cerebral blood flow.

Emergency treatment is not necessary for recovery is spontaneous. Therapy directed to the prevention of future attacks will not be discussed here.

Valsalva maneuver Fainting due to a strong Valsalva maneuver resembles that of cough syncope. There is a similar obstruction to the entrance of blood into the thorax; at the same time the heart may be compressed. The diminished inflow and this compression in turn induce a fall in the effective output of the heart and in the level of systemic blood pressure. As in gardener's syncope, to be described later, there may be a further fall in systemic blood pressure on release of the maneuver. And it is at this time that the subject may faint. "Blackouts" or deaths on the bedpan, death during post-operative tracheal suction and "micturition syncope" probably have a like mechanism. The latter condition has already been mentioned under nitroglycerin collapse (p. 56). Its occurrence suggests unusually severe straining and may be a clue to the existence of prostatism.

CARDIAC SYNCOPE

Syncope may occur in association with disturbances in rhythm or conduction or in aortic stenosis. With these notable exceptions fainting is not a common symptom of heart disease. Syncope is almost unheard of in congestive heart failure. This has been explained by the elevation in the venous pressure [2]

and constant vasoconstriction: only under exceptional circumstances would venous pressure be reduced sufficiently to precipitate a faint. It is principally at the onset of a paroxysm of
rapid heart action, be it atrial tachycardia, flutter or fibrillation
or ventricular tachycardia, when the cardiovascular apparatus
is overwhelmed and compensatory mechanisms have not yet
become effective that fainting occurs. During ventricular fibrillation or during the so-called "post-undulatory pause" that
follows ventricular tachycardia, syncope may also occur. These
tachysystoles are fully discussed in Chapters 9 through 13.
Syncope, of course, is the presenting symptom of Adams-Stokes
attacks (Chapter 14). It is not generally appreciated that
fainting can also occur during intermissions of the heart beat,
due to sino-atrial block or sinus pauses, and the consequent
fall in systemic blood pressure. These intervals of cardiac
standstill can last as long as, and produce the same symptoms
as those of Adams-Stokes attacks. During sinus pauses one
fails to hear heart sounds and the electrocardiogram demon-
strates lack of atrial or ventricular activity. After several seconds
(4 to 8 seconds if the patient is standing, 6 to 10 seconds if
sitting, and 12 to 15 seconds if recumbent),[8] of cardiac quiescence the patient loses consciousness. If the pause continues he
may convulse. Such periods of standstill may occur as the effer-
ent effect of a reflex arc in which such diverse conditions as
carotid sinus sensitivity, gall bladder disease, esophageal or duodenal diverticulum, mediastinal carcinoma, a mass pressing
upon the carotid sinus or vagus nerve, cardiospasm, broncho-
scopic examination, or even diseased tonsils stimulate the effer-
ent arc. Immediate treatment consists of atropine or ephedrine
in full therapeutic dosage. For persistent and repetitive attacks
a probable or suspected reflex focus may have to be removed.
In severe cases with recurrent or prolonged periods of asystole
one may have to employ those measures which are ordinarily
used for Adams-Stokes attacks, including epinephrine, isopropyl

arterenol and the cardiac pacemaker. In certain instances denervation of the carotid sinus has been practiced, with an occasional reported success.

Syncope in aortic stenosis is generally preceded by a brief period of dizziness. This frequently lasts long enough to give the patient time to ease himself into a position in which he will not fall when he loses consciousness. Furthermore syncope may not occur unless a certain level of exertion is exceeded.[21] Accordingly it is rare for these patients to suffer injury with their syncopal attacks. The heart rate is slow and can be accelerated but little, systole is prolonged and the cardiac output relatively fixed. Apparently there is no uniform mechanism in the syncopal episodes. They are commonly explained by a temporary failure of the left ventricle to empty itself satisfactorily. But it is more likely that the explanation is transient peripheral vasodilatation; with fixed heart rate and cardiac output incapable of increasing adequately, this vaso-motor reaction diverts blood from brain to periphery. I have seen a number of patients with aortic stenosis in whom carotid sinus stimulation induced cardiac slowing. In others paroxysmal rapid heart action such as atrial fibrillation triggered syncope. But these are the exception rather than the rule.

Syncope is an ominous development in aortic stenosis and often the forerunner of a sudden fatality. In view of this unpredictability and of the improvement in the results of aortic valve surgery, serious consideration should be given to the advisability of surgical repair of the stenosed aortic valve.

On rare occasions syncope occurs at the onset of acute myocardial infarction. It is probably related to the severity of the pain in these cases for extreme pain from other causes may do the same thing. The mechanism of the syncope is probably similar to that of the simple faint as described on page 314. Treatment consists of relief of pain.

Syncope may be induced by the engagement of a *ball valve*

thrombus or a *pedunculated myxoma* or *sarcoma* of the left atrium into the mitral valve orifice. A clue to these conditions may be the abrupt development of syncope or dyspnea in patients with real or presumed mitral stenosis on change of posture. Return to consciousness may also be abrupt and complete. Occasionally the murmur of mitral stenosis may be made to come and go by deliberately changing the patient's position, but this may be difficult to evaluate for the murmur may thus be made to change in intensity or to disappear for other reasons. A tumor or thrombus may first be suspected during left heart catheterization and demonstrated more certainly by angiocardiography. Sometimes it is first detected during surgery for repair of the mitral valve, definitive surgery being done at a subsequent operation.

Syncope or lesser cerebral symptoms such as dizziness may be the presenting complaint in *pulmonary embolism*. The management of this condition is detailed in Chapter 5.

Fainting may also occur in certain forms of cyanotic (e.g. Tetralogy of Fallot) or acyanotic (e.g. congenital subaortic stenosis) *congenital heart disease*. In both of these sub-groups, exertion seems to play a determining rôle in the precipitation of syncope. In the cyanotic group, exercise increases the volume of right-to-left blood flow across the shunt and thus the degree of arterial oxygen unsaturation—this then is an example of so-called "anoxic syncope." Oxygen is of limited value for it cannot correct arterial unsaturation which is due to a shunt. In infants and children, pushing the knees into the chest, as in the squatting position, or, in adults, the knee chest position, may relieve the symptoms attributable to pronounced hypoxemia. Opinion is not unanimous on how this improvement is brought about. Some attribute it to decreased, others to increased venous return, and still others to increased systemic resistance. In other defects diverse mechanisms may be involved; in congenital sub-aortic stenosis this is probably similar

[325]

to that of acquired aortic stenosis. There is no immediate treatment since the activity which precipitates syncope necessarily stops at the moment of syncope. In all of these congenital cardiac defects thought will be given to the feasibility of corrective cardiac surgery.

CEREBRAL SYNCOPE

Syncope is often the manifestation of cerebral vascular insufficiency. Often it is accompanied or followed by evanescent focal neurological findings. If syncope results from cerebral hemorrhage, and the hemorrhage from hypertension, it is expected that hypertension will be detectable even after the faint. If hypertension is not present, particularly in young or middle-aged persons, consideration should be given to the possibility of ruptured aneurysm, meningo-vascular syphilis, polycythemia, carotid artery thrombosis or hemorrhage into a brain tumor. Bland cerebral embolism from mural atrial thrombi in mitral stenosis or atrial fibrillation, from mural thrombi in acute or subacute myocardial infarction, or ventricular aneurysm or from infected vegetations in bacterial endocarditis, or nonspecific endomyocarditis must all be thought of.

Acute crises of *hypertensive encephalopathy* may punctuate the course of hypertensive cardiovascular disease particularly in that period of rapidly advancing symptomatology which is commonly designated as malignant hypertension. In these patients the transient hemiplegia, monoplegia, aphasia, blindness or syncope is often preceded by a brief rise in the level of the blood pressure. In this situation prompt relief of the dangerously elevated pressure is mandatory. This is effected by the infusion of Arfonad as described on page 34 or by the intramuscular injection of 2.5 to 5.0 mgm. of reserpine given at intervals of 6 to 12 hours, dosage and interval being de-

[326]

termined by the blood pressure response.[22] An effect is not to be expected until an hour or two after the injection. If this does not control the symptoms or the blood pressure, recourse may be had to the intravenous use of the veratrum drugs. In general one should attempt a gradual rather than an abrupt lowering of the blood pressure level.

There is often considerable difficulty in distinguishing *epileptiform seizures* from syncope due to the various cardiovascular abnormalities thus far considered. Certain features of the attack point toward epilepsy as its cause.[23] In an attack, the previously untreated patient becomes rigid, falls and exhibits some form of clonic or tonic movement. The skin is commonly florid or cyanotic, rarely pale, it may feel hot and damp, or cool and dry but rarely if ever cool and damp. Unconsciousness is commonly preceded by visual, olfactory or motor aura; these don't occur in syncope due to other causes. In epilepsy the patient falls "hard;" muscle tone increases, the body stiffens and the patient characteristically topples like an upset statue. In other forms of syncope he slumps. In epilepsy the patient may bite his tongue or lips and wet or soil himself. In the majority of cases the attacks are followed by drowsiness, headache or sleep ("post-ictal state"). Neurological examination immediately after an attack may show a Babinski sign. The emergency treatment is the prevention of injury to the patient, inserting a mouth gag, loosening the collar, and providing an adequate airway perhaps simply by holding his chin forward.

Hysterical syncope may also be confused with syncope due to cardiovascular mechanisms. This form of syncope does not occur at inopportune times as when the patient is alone. These commonly appear following a rebuff or when the patient feels it is important to attract attention. During the attack the eyes are closed and the patient resists any attempt to open them. The attack may last longer than any of the conditions thus far described. The fall is soft and unassociated with injury or incontinence. Neurological examination after the attack is negative. Diagnosis is often difficult. Treatment is psychiatric in approach: there is no emergency medical therapy.

Multiple mechanisms are not uncommon and may reinforce the tendency to syncope. Many people faint because they have underlying cerebral vascular sclerosis or stenosis which seems to potentiate or make manifest any of the mechanisms described above. Hypoglycemia and carotid sinus sensitivity seem to enhance one another. The same applies to hypoglycemia and the hyperventilation syndrome.[24] A syncopal reaction is much more likely to develop when there is already a pronounced vasodilatation as on a hot day or after a soaking hot tub bath. "Gardener's syncope" is apparently due in the first place to a squeezing of blood out of the leg veins on squatting. This increases cardiac filling pressure, stroke output and pulse pressure. This in turn leads to a baroreceptor vasodilatation. The sudden assumption of the erect posture now causes an abrupt fall in filling pressure and cardiac output while vasodilatation is still present. There may be a few seconds therefore before vasoconstriction is effective, when syncope may occur.[2]

REFERENCES

(1) Lewis, T.: A lecture on vasovagal syncope and the carotid sinus syndrome. With comments on Gowers' and Nothnagel's syndrome. Brit. Med. J. 1: 873, 1932.

(2) Sharpey-Schafer, E. P.: Emergencies in general practice. Syncope. Brit. Med. J. 1: 506, 1956.

(3) Weiss, S. and Baker, J. P.: The carotid sinus reflex in health and disease. Its rôle in the causation of fainting and convulsion. Medicine, 12: 297, 1933.

(4) Ferris, E. B., Capps, R. B. and Weiss, S.: Carotid sinus syndrome and its bearing on the mechanism of the unconscious state and convulsions. Medicine, 14: 377, 1955.

(5) Heymans, C. and Neil, E.: Reflexogenic Areas of the Cardiovascular System. Little Brown and Company, Boston, 1958.

(6) Friedberg, C. K.: Diseases of the Heart. W. B. Saunders, Philadelphia and London. Second Edition, 1956, p. 312.

(7) Ray, B. S. and Stewart, H. J.: Rôle of the glossopharyngeal nerve in the carotid sinus reflex in man. Surgery 23: 411, 1948.

(8) Engel, G. L.: Fainting. Physiological and Psychological Considerations. Charles C. Thomas, Springfield, Illinois, 1950, p. 75.

(9) Lewis, B. I.: The hyperventilation syndrome. Ann. Int. Med. 38: 918, 1953.

(10) Ellis, L. B.. and Haynes, F.: Postural hypotension, with particular reference to its occurrence in disease of the central nervous system. Arch. Int. Med. 58: 773, 1936.

(11) Smithwick, R. H., Kinsey, D. and Whitelow, G. T.: A screening test for adrenal or unilateral renal forms of hypertension based upon postural changes in blood pressure. Read at annual meeting of American Heart Association. October, 1957.

(12) Sieker, H. O., Barnum, J. F., Hickam, J. B. and Penrod, K. E.: Treatment of postural hypotension with counterpressure garment. J.A.M.A. 161: 132, 1956.

(13) Gregory, R.: The treatment of orthostatic hypotension. With particular reference to the use of desoxycorticosterone. Am. Ht. J. 29: 246, 1945.

(14) Hickler, R. B., Thompson, G. R., Fox, L. M. and Hamlin, J. T. III: Successful treatment of orthostatic hypotension with 9-alphafluorocortisone. N.E.J. Med. 261: 788, 1959.

(15) Ebert, R. V., Stead, E. A., Jr. and Gibson, J. G. III: Response of normal subjects to acute blood loss. Arch. Int. Med. 68: 578, 1941.

(16) Edwards, E. A.: Varicose veins and venous stasis. Bolet-

in de la Association Medice de Puerto Rico, 49: 49, 1957.

(17) Levine, H. D.: Urticaria due to sensitivity to cold. Arch. Int. Med. 56: 498, 1935.

(18) Affolter, J.: Urticaria et syncope "a frigore." Schweiz. med. Wchnschr. 63: 881, 1933.

(19) Kerr, A., Jr. and Derbes, V. J.: The syndrome of cough syncope. Ann. Int. Med. 39: 1240, 1953.

(20) Wood, P.: Diseases of the Heart and Circulation. J. B. Lippincott Co., Second Edition, 1956, p. 17.

(21) Contratto, A. W. and Levine, S. A.: Aortic stenosis with special reference to angina pectoris and syncope. Ann. Int. Med. 10: 1636, 1937.

(22) Meilman, E.: The treatment of hypertension. Medical Science. J. B. Lippincott, Philadelphia. 6: 789, 1959.

(23) Ives, E. R.: Epileptic seizures differentiated from cardio-vascular syncope and functional episodes. J.A.M. Women's Ass'n. 13: 226, 1958.

(24) Engel, G. L., Ferris, E. B. and Logan, B.: Hyperventilation: analysis of clinical symptomatology. Ann. Int. Med. 27: 683, 1947.

16

CARDIAC ARREST AND

RESUSCITATION

The Anticipated or Imminent Emergency

Recognition of Cardiac Arrest

Management of Ventricular Standstill

Procedure for Ventricular Fibrillation

16

CARDIAC ARREST AND

RESUSCITATION

It goes almost without saying that any non-beating heart may be considered a heart in arrest. Thus whatever the initiating mechanism, whether ventricular fibrillation or primary ventricular inhibition, and whether due to coronary occlusion, to pulmonary embolism or to exsanguination, the end result must be standstill or arrest of the heart. But, as ordinarily understood, the term "cardiac arrest" has the further implication of reversibility; though electrical and mechanical activity have ceased, the heart can be aroused and a normal cardiac mechanism resumed. An "arrested" heart then, is not a dead heart. Unfortunately the term has come to have different meanings to different people. The internist or cardiologist thinks of "cardiac arrest" primarily as a cardiac inhibition whether from the toxic effects of certain drugs such as digitalis, quinidine or procaine amide or from changes in the electrolyte composition of blood or myocardium (e.g. potassium intoxication or potassium depletion) or from extreme vagal inhibition such as might be implemented by an active vago-vagal reflex. Or it might be the mechanism of an Adams-Stokes attack. To the internist it is not necessary that this event be related to surgery. The surgeon, on the other hand, thinks of cardiac arrest as an acute unexpected cessation of cardiac activity occurring during or after operation (not necessarily major surgery), during the induction of, or emergence from, anaesthesia and during certain procedures such as intubation of the trachea. In the view of some [1] it may be the concerted effect of a few, or of many, of a multitude of abnormal physiological processes including hypoxia, hypercapnia, hypovolemia, excessive anaesthetic agent, careless transfer of or positioning of the patient, electrolyte disturbances, etc.

THE ANTICIPATED OR IMMINENT EMERGENCY

Certain groups of patients are much more vulnerable than others to standstill or fibrillation of the ventricles during anaesthesia or surgery. This includes patients undergoing intracranial, thoracic or cardiac surgery, those in whom hypothermia has been utilized, extremely debilitated patients, individuals with potassium intoxication or hyperkalemia, those with sensitivity of the carotid sinus, patients who have already demonstrated attacks of paroxysmal ventricular tachycardia, cardiac arrest or ventricular fibrillation and, most frequent of all, patients with severe heart disease, especially coronary artery disease, valvular heart disease (and more particularly those with the combination of coronary disease and aortic stenosis), atrioventricular block of any degree and patients receiving quinidine or procaine amide. Patients are also vulnerable who have been maintained on some of the newer drugs such as the steroids, thorazine, the tranquilizing agents and the hypotensive agents (such as serpasil). These matters cannot be ignored by the surgeon or anaesthetist. Drugs of the latter two categories ought therefore to be discontinued two weeks or so before anticipated surgery. The internist owes it to surgeon and anaesthetist to let them know what drugs the patient has been

[334]

and is receiving,[2] but this does not absolve the anaesthetist of the responsibility of making every effort to find out about previous and current medication. A perfectly normal heart can also develop "arrest;" there is reason to believe that this occurs only when hypoxia is coupled with vagal depression.[3] But the overwhelming majority of "arrests" develop in "good risk" patients because of overdose of anaesthetic agent.

Since this event is a potential occurrence in any patient undergoing anaesthesia or surgery, it is imperative that both anaesthetist and surgeon be constantly alert to detect the brady-cardia and hypotension that commonly herald cardiac arrest. In the average case the usual careful monitoring of pulse and blood pressure, especially during induction, tracheal intubation and changing of the patient's position will suffice. In the specially vulnerable patients enumerated above, monitoring with the electrocardiogram or cardioscope should be added. Probably the most sensitive index of impending arrest is the two-lead electroencephalogram. Decreased cerebral oxygenation is observable with this instrument much earlier than are changes in the electrocardiogram.

Though anaesthetics commonly mask all circulatory and respiratory signs of hypoxia and hypercarbia, the development of cardiac arrest during anaesthesia and operation can often be anticipated by the alert anaesthetist. The premonitory signs which presage this catastrophe are those of asphyxia and include cyanosis, transient tachycardia and elevation of blood pressure. These generally precede the more ominous development of bradycardia and hypotension.[3] Cardia arrhythmias, sweating, changes in skin color and changes in the pattern of breathing may also portend impending disaster.[1] There are several more advanced signs indicating collapse: a weak, barely perceptible pulse, a weak pulsation in a major artery, pupillary dilatation, little or no active bleeding, an unobtainable blood pressure and the development of pallor of the skin. But I think it is fair to say that, even in the hands of the most competent, cardiac arrest, though never unexpected, often appears completely unheralded; this concession does not condone the least departure from constant vigilance on the part of surgeon and anaesthetist.

If the danger of impending arrest is recognized at this time, certain corrective steps may yet forestall actual standstill. The patient's lungs should be ventilated immediately and vigorously with oxygen and the patient should be given an infusion of neosynephrine or nor-epinephrine as outlined on page 42. The orthopneic cardiac patient who has carelessly been allowed to lie flat should have his head and chest elevated. If the patient has not already received an injection of atropine, this should be given forthwith by vein in the dose of o.4 to o.6 mgm. to interrupt a possible vago-vagal reflex. This must be done carefully; atropine given in large doses or large increments may have prominent vagal effects and induce, rather than prevent, collapse. Where feasible the intramuscular route is preferred.

One must insure a clear airway by proper positioning of the head and neck and, if obstruction is still present, by the insertion of an endotracheal airway and the removal with suction of secretions, blood or aspirated bowel fluid. Where the use of the endotracheal tube is impossible it may be necessary to perform a tracheotomy. During thoracic surgery compression or displacement of the heart, lung, and great vessels or distortion of their relationships by retractors or packs must be recognized and corrected. The infusion system should be checked for clotting in the apparatus and injection sites for paravenous injection. If blood is given under pressure one must be certain that the reservoir is not empty and that air has not been injected.

RECOGNITION OF CARDIAC ARREST

Certain changes indicate that arrest is not merely imminent but actually at hand: a peripheral pulse, known previously to have been present, cannot be felt at all; the blood pressure cannot be obtained with the sphygmomanometer; there is no active bleeding whatever; the color of the skin becomes waxy; the pupils are dilated; and breathing occurs in apneustic gasps. Immediate action is mandatory. Any of these findings should be regarded as presumptive evidence of cardiac arrest, but they can also be noted in peripheral vascular collapse. This presumptive diagnosis can be confirmed in a number of ways. The anaesthetist fails to feel a carotid artery pulsation or the surgeon to feel the pulsation of the aorta. The heart sounds are not heard or the heart movements felt. And if a monitoring device is running normal electrocardiographic complexes are generally not recorded. The operation, even though incomplete, is discontinued at once. Certainly at this point one should not lose time to attach and record an electrocardiogram. An un-attached stethoscope can be of inestimable value in the operating room at this time. There should always be one on the anaesthetist's table; every anaesthetist should carry one. The absence of heart sounds is very good evidence of standstill.

Let us assume that the surgeon has satisfied himself that there is no peripheral blood flow; he must now make a quick decision. He is confronted with a 95% probability of cardiac standstill and a 5% possibility of ventricular fibrillation as the underlying mechanism. He will already have thought through a point of view in relation to this hypothetical and actual situation. The surgical team, surgeon and anaesthetist, will already have rehearsed repeatedly with firedrill precision, just what is to be done. All necessary equipment must be at hand and in working order. There is not time to make up the necessary solutions. A special emergency tray should be available con-

[337]

taining scalpel, 1:1000 epinephrine solution, 10% calcium chloride solution and 1% procaine hydrochloride solution.

MANAGEMENT OF VENTRICULAR STANDSTILL

The duties of the surgical team and the anaesthetic team will be concurrent and coordinated. (See Charts I and II.) The surgeon should pause to thump the chest. In rare cases this may restart the heartbeat. Or the heart may be stimulated through the intact chest wall with the tip of a needle. If the abdomen is open he should strike a blow to the heart through the diaphragm. If these maneuvers are unsuccessful—and they generally are—one proceeds immediately to enter the chest without bothering about asepsis.

In the meantime the anaesthetist has discontinued anaesthesia, has lowered the patient into a slight Trendelenburg position, and has immediately started artificial respiration. In the operating room this is done with a face mask or through an endotracheal tube, the bag being flushed repeatedly with 100% oxygen. If this is not feasible, mouth-to-mouth breathing is employed. Forgetting all aesthetics and with his wide-opened mouth closely applied about the patient's open mouth, and the patient's jaw held upward and forward, and neck fully extended the anaesthetist breathes rhythmically into the patient's mouth. He ensures that ventilation is adequate by observing ample excursion of the patient's chest. On removal of the physician's mouth from that of the patient, expiration occurs passively. A refinement of this technique is the use of the double-ended oropharyngeal tube (Fig. 41). At the same time a pre-arranged member of the surgical team, generally a medical student or nurse, has recorded the time when arrest was first noted and keeps a time record of all procedures, drugs and responses.

An incision is made from the sternum to the mid-axillary

CHART I. RESTORATION OF SPONTANEOUS HEART BEAT

Once adequate manual systole has been established proceed deliberately but *DO NOT INTERRUPT MANUAL SYSTOLE, OR CONTINUOUS VIGOROUS VENTILATION.* Do not wait to intubate; use face mask. Mouth to mouth breathing only if proper equipment unavailable. Resuscitation has been effective even after 2 or more hours of manual systole.

A. *Ventricular Standstill:*

1) If standstill persists after 3 minutes of manual systole, inject diluted epinephrine into left atrial chamber. (Dilute 1 cc 1:1000 epinephrine in 10 cc; inject 1 cc initially and repeat in 3 minutes if necessary.)

2) If arrest continues and myocardium is flabby, inject 5 cc of 10% calcium chloride into left atrial chamber.

3) Electric pacemaker applied directly to ventricle (80/min at 15 volts or less) may evoke effective beats.

B. *Ventricular Fibrillation:*

1) Manual systole must be continued until myocardium is pink and firm. An anoxic heart cannot be defibrillated.

2) Then, electric shock defibrillation (60 cycle A-C; 0.05 second at 280 volts). Compress heart between large electrodes to prevent spark burns and apply single shock. If necessary, use 2 shocks at 1-second intervals.

PRECAUTIONS: Avoid direct contact between electrodes and contact with operator. After resuscitation, repeated arrest can recur. Consider continuous ECG monitor; cardiac pacemaker should be available.

CHART II. TREATMENT OF CARDIAC ARREST

Circulation of oxygenated blood should be restored within 2 minutes

DO NOT WAIT FOR ELECTROCARDIOGRAM

SIMULTANEOUS ACTION

ANAESTHETIST

1. Stop anaesthesia.
2. Ventilate vigorously with pure oxygen (flush bag repeatedly).
3. Clear airway; oral airway and face mask or endotracheal tube.
4. Designate recorder to note time of arrest, procedures, drugs and responses.
5. Evaluate circulation. Manual systole and ventilation are inadequate if pupils remain dilated, cyanosis persists, carotid pulse is absent.

SURGEON

1. Stop operation.
2. *Mechanical stimulation.* Blow to ｜ cordium or needle puncture of hea If abdomen is open, stimulate acr diaphragm.
3. *External electric stimulation* with ｜ diac pacemaker *if attached.*

IF NOT IMMEDIATELY EFFF TIVE:

4. *Manual systole.* Rapid thoracotc (4th or 5th left intercostal) with delay for asepsis. Forceful but ge｜ manual systole 60/min. Insert spreader, open pericardium, occl｜ descending aorta if necessary.
5. *Confirm adequacy* of manual syst with anaesthetist.

Modification of Guide prepared by Committee on Cardiac Arrest, Massachusett Heart Association.[5]

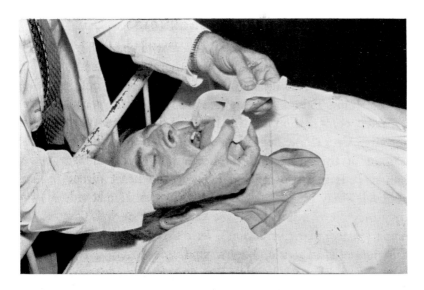

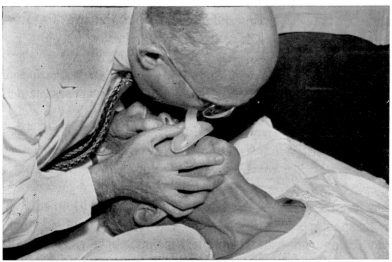

Fig. 41. *Mouth-to-mouth Breathing with Double-ended Resuscitator Tube.*
Above: The oropharyngeal tube is inserted with patient's head hyperextended
and tongue held forward with gauze pad. Below: Method of artificial respiration.
Chin held forward, head hyperextended, nostrils held shut. The physician
breathes regularly and rhythmically into the tube at about 10 to 12 times per
minute, checking adequacy of expansion of patient's chest with each breath
and ensuring that patient pinks up properly. Expiration is passive. If tube is
not available this may be accomplished similarly by direct mouth-to-mouth
breathing.

[341]

line along the fourth or fifth left intercostal space. This should require less than 30 seconds since there is no bleeding. The pericardium is next opened, taking care not to cut into the myocardium. This takes only a few seconds and permits more effective compression of the heart and a better view of its activity. A rib retractor is placed in position to facilitate manipulation of the heart and minimize fatigue of the surgeon's hands. It is now possible to observe the heart directly. The ventricles may be completely quiescent (cardiac standstill) or they may show a fine or coarse undulatory or writhing movement (ventricular fibrillation). In either case, the surgeon, at the patient's left side, begins rhythmic compression of the ventricles with both hands (Fig. 42), taking care not to perforate the myocardium with undue pressure of any finger or thumb. Manual systole should be kept up at the rate of at least 60 times per minute. Effective systole is checked by palpation of the carotid or radial artery or by an effective rise in blood pressure. If a pulse cannot be felt or the pupils remain dilated, manual compression is inadequate and more vigorous manual systole and compression of the descending aorta are in order. When this emergency arises during an abdominal operation some authorities advise attempting repeated compression of the heart against the back of the sternum through the intact diaphragm. This rarely gives an effective output and should not be persisted in if the heart does not respond immediately with spontaneous beating. With the restoration of adequate ventilation and manual systole the immediate emergency is over.

It may be wise now to prepare and drape the skin and to have the first surgeon or another surgeon substitute an aseptic technique. It is truly surprising how rarely infection has complicated recovery in these cases despite the lack of initial asepsis. I know of one individual whose chest was opened in the manner described above on the contaminated floor of an

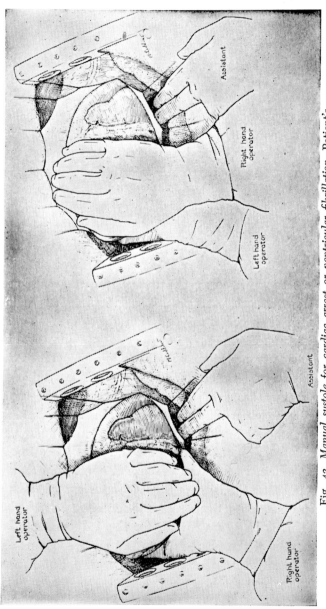

Fig. 42. *Manual systole for cardiac arrest or ventricular fibrillation.* Patient's head to right, feet to left of operative field. Pericardium opened. The ventricles are rhythmically emptied by firm but gentle compression with both hands. Fatigue is minimized by periodically changing the relative position of the hands. (Drawings by Mildred B. Codding)

experimental laboratory but who failed to develop any evidence of sepsis. If possible the descending aorta should be occluded. After a few minutes of continued compression one may pause to observe whether spontaneous cardiac contractions have started. If the heart remains in standstill, compression is resumed and the heart observed periodically for spontaneous beating. So long as the "tone" of the heart remains firm this process may be continued for long periods of time, hours if necessary, avoiding fatigue by changing the relative position of the hands (Fig. 42) or by periodic spelling of the person carrying out manual systole. If standstill persists after three minutes of manual compression or the heart seems to lack "tone," one may inject 5 cc. of diluted epinephrine solution (1 cc. of 1:1000 epinephrine added to 9 cc. of dextrose and water solution) into the left atrial chamber.[5] Before this injection is given one must be certain that the heart is pink else epinephrine may induce ventricular fibrillation. If this is ineffective one injects 5 cc. of 10% solution of calcium chloride into the left atrium. Or one may try 50 cc. of 50% dextrose in water. Finally 0.02 to 0.04 mgm. of isopropyl-norepinephrine in 10 cc. of dextrose and water should be tried. The sympathico-mometic amines are said to have the paradoxical effect of initiating ventricular fibrillation in large doses but of preventing or antagonizing it in small dosage. Manual compression is continued throughout these procedures. If these injections are not followed by return of normal contractions they may be repeated after the lapse of three minutes or so. It is difficult to define just when these resuscitative efforts should be abandoned. This is largely a matter for the judgment of the surgeon. Generally if the heart fails to resume a spontaneous beat after an hour further efforts are unsuccessful. But I have seen patients in whom the heart has revived after longer periods. When the tone of the heart remains firm and when the initial period of standstill before undertaking manual systole

[344]

has been less than four minutes, one will be encouraged to more persistent efforts. When the heart is relaxed, on the other hand, and when the period of standstill exceeded four minutes, one will be less sanguine about their worthwhileness. Although it is commonly stated that there is a critical period of four minutes beyond which irreversible cerebral damage necessarily follows [8,9], I have seen a number of patients in whom the probable duration of arrested cerebral circulation exceeded four minutes, yet recovery was without detectable cerebral residual.

PROCEDURE FOR VENTRICULAR FIBRILLATION

When, on entering the chest the ventricles are found to be fibrillating, the "tone" of the heart may still be strong and its color pink; but when fibrillation has lasted some time the ventricles are apt to be soft, purple and dilated. In either case the treatment is that used for standstill, namely rhythmic manual compression. This may improve the tone of the relaxed heart but it is generally not adequate to convert the heart from fibrillation to standstill. Where fibrillation persists, continued compression can maintain an adequate cerebral and coronary circulation until more specific defibrillatory measures can be employed. One of these is the use of an electrical defibrillator. This consists of a pair of large metal plates which are applied one to the anterior surface and the other to the posterior surface of the heart, extending close to the apex,[10] and across which an electroshock of more than 220 volts with a duration of 0.1 second or less can be delivered. Amperage will depend upon the mass of myocardium. One should avoid direct contact between electrodes. And it is best to have saline soaked gauze pads between the electrodes and the epicardium to improve contact. Personnel must take careful precautions to avoid direct or indirect contact with the defibrillator. At first one may deliver a single shock.[11,12] If this is ineffective in stopping the fibrillation two may be given in rapid succession. Whether or not the fibrillation has been stopped, manual compression must be resumed promptly after shocking. If the electrical defibrillator is ineffective, defibrillation may be attempted by chemical means. For this purpose 6–8 milliequivalents of potassium chloride should be injected into the root of the aorta while the aorta is briefly occluded distally and manual systole is continued. If this is unsuccessful one may inject 10 cc. of 1% solution of procaine hydrochloride into the left atrium. Much has been made of the need to wash out the injected potassium salts with other solutions once fibrillation has been converted to standstill, but it seems probable that manual compression alone is effective in dissipating this from the myocardium. The objection has been raised that either of these agents, potassium or procaine, can theoretically depress an already depressed myocardium. The validity of this objection in this situation has not been determined. Once fibrillation has been stopped, the surgeon proceeds with the management of standstill as outlined above.

After successful resuscitation, arrest or fibrillation may recur. The heart should therefore be monitored continuously with the electrocardiograph during closure and recovery. Continued oxygenation is most important and, if the blood pressure is low, pressor amines should be continued. At this juncture it is well to have an external "pacemaker" attached and ready for use and an external defibrillator at hand. The application of an external pacemaker or defibrillator at the outset of this operating room emergency is out of the question. Used in the event of a recurrent episode there would seem to be a better rationale for the applicability of either, since the appropriate technique would then be available for immediate use. If recurrence has not been anticipated, one should not waste time to attach the external apparatus but should proceed immediately to re-open the chest. The use of the external pacemaker [14,15] has been de-

[346]

scribed on p. 301. The external defibrillator,[15,16] which likewise is used across the unopened chest, consists of a pair of large copper electrodes 7.5 cms. in diameter, which are coated with electrode paste and held in place, one to the left of the sternum and the other in the anterior axillary line, and across which varying voltages are impressed at a current of 15 amperes for 0.15 second at a time. The voltage is varied from 120 to 720 volts by means of a step-up transformer and a variable autotransformer. During the application of this very high voltage the electrocardiograph machine or Cardioscope must be turned off. And the attending physicians must be warned against touching the electrodes or the patient during the shock. If ineffective at lower electromotive force the voltage can be increased stepwise at intervals of several seconds. Once standstill has successfully been attained an attempt is made to restore a normal sinus mechanism with the use of the external pacemaker. Either technique may be worth a single try under the circumstances assuming that the apparatus is already attached and ready for use, but, if ineffective, one should abandon the external approach at once, promptly re-open the chest and deal with the situation as outlined above.

If resuscitative efforts of this type are not only justifiable but mandatory in the operating room, may they not also be employed elsewhere? Is salvage possible, for example, in any considerable number of patients with heart disease whose heart action suddenly and unexpectedly stops? In those patients in whom ventricular fibrillation or ventricular standstill seems destined to be their terminal mechanism, is it not possible that abolition of this disturbance may yet save the patient's life and allow him to survive for a longer or shorter period? An answer to these questions based on actual experience is not available. A partial answer is provided in the experimental observations of Wiggers[11] who found that coronary artery ligation in dogs induces ventricular fibrillation, that this can be abolished by electric shock but that fibrillation recurs promptly unless the ligature about the coronary branch is loosened. This seems to furnish a clue that ventricular fibrillation occurring in the course of acute myocardial infarction, even if abolished, would be likely to recur; the cessation of the heart beat must then be the inexorable result of advanced and irreversible disease. But, in the opinion of some, the appearance of many of these hearts at post-mortem has been judged as capable of long survival if only the heart could be made to survive the acute arrhythmia. While accepting this formulation in principle one cannot help but feel that a decision on whether such a heart can be revived may be beyond the competency of most humans. As yet no clear-cut criteria have been established to indicate when attempts at "death reversal" are justified. It would only be by lucky chance, furthermore, that the diagnosis might be made in time [16,17] and that a prepared physician would be at hand to start appropriate therapy promptly. But already a half dozen cases or so have been reported in which thoracotomy has been carried out for ventricular arrest or fibrillation during acute myocardial infarction and the heart successfully resuscitated. Since we are not so prone to report our failures, there is no way of knowing how many unsuccessful attempts have been made. Wholesale, indiscriminate thoracotomy in patients who have just died of acute myocardial infarction is to be condemned. It could become a ghastly ritual and place the whole rationale and practice of this procedure into disrepute. Until more experience has been accumulated it is suggested that thoracotomy and manual systole are ill-advised when the patient is outside of a hospital, when acute myocardial infarction, or pulmonary embolism is obvious, or when cardiac arrest is a terminal event after a protracted illness, after a long period of shock or after severe sepsis or trauma.

One could be more enthusiastic about, or less disinclined to, bloodless efforts at reviving such patients with the external pacemaker [14,15] or defibrillator.[15,16] It has been suggested that there should be one of each on every medical and surgical floor.

REFERENCES

(1) Natof, H. E. and Sadove, M. S.: Cardiovascular Collapse in the Operating Room. J. B. Lippincott Co., Philadelphia and Montreal, 1958.
(2) Vandam, L. D.: Personal communication.
(3) Effler, D. B. and Sifers, E. C.: Cardiac arrest. Cleveland Clinic Quarterly, *19*: 194, 1952.
(4) Kasler, M. H., Frye, C. W. and Gordon, A. S.: Postural hypotension induced by atropine sulfate. Circulation *10*: 413, 1954.
(5) Zoll, P. M., Friedlich, A. L., Harken, D. E., Hegnauer, A. H. and Nicholson, M. J.: Cardiac arrest. Summary of its management developed by Committee on Cardiac Arrest. Massachusetts Heart Association, 1957.
(6) Adams, H. D. and Hand, L. V.: Twenty minute cardiac arrest with complete recovery. J.A.M.A. *118*: 133, 1943.
(7) Carter, M. G.: Cardiac arrest. Complete recovery after twenty-five minutes. J.A.M.A. *147*: 1347, 1951.
(8) Weinberger, L. M., Gibbon, M. H. and Gibbon, J. H., Jr.: Temporary arrest of circulation to central nervous system. I. Physiologic effects. Arch. Neurol. and Psychiat. *43*: 615, 1940.
(9) Cole, S. L. and Corday, E.: Four-minute limit for cardiac resuscitation. J.A.M.A. *161*: 1454, 1956.
(10) Bigelow, W. C., Heimbecker, R. O. and Thrusler, G.: The practical management of cardiac arrest. Canad. Med. Ass'n. J. *76*: 86, 1957.
(11) Wiggers, C. J.: The physiologic basis for cardiac resus-

citation from ventricular fibrillation—Method for serial defibrillation. Am. Ht. J. 20: 413, 1940.

(12) Leeds, S. E.: Cardiac resuscitation. J.A.M.A. 152: 1409, 1953.

(13) Dripps, R. D., Eckenhoff, J. E. and Vandam, L. D.: Introduction to Anaesthesia. The Principles of Safe Practice. W. B. Saunders Co., Philadelphia and London, 1957, p. 208.

(14) Zoll, P. M.: Resuscitation of the heart in ventricular standstill by external electric stimulation. N.E.J. Med. 247: 768, 1952.

(15) Zoll, P. M., Linenthal, A. J., Norman, L. R., Paul, M. H. and Gibson, W.: External electric stimulation of heart in cardiac arrest. Arch. Int. Med. 96: 639, 1955.

(16) Zoll, P. M., Linenthal, A. J., Gibson, W., Paul, M. H. and Norman, L. R.: Termination of ventricular fibrillation in man by externally applied electric countershock. N.E.J. Med. 254: 727, 1956.

(17) Mozen, H. E., Katzman, R. and Martin, J. W.: Successful defibrillation of the heart. Resuscitative procedure started on medical ward and completed in operating room. J.A.M.A. 162: 111, 1956.

CHAPTER

17

MISCELLANEOUS

EMERGENCIES

Pericardial Tamponade

Venous Air Embolism

Fat Embolism

17

MISCELLANEOUS

EMERGENCIES

In the present chapter a few conditions are considered which do not quite properly fall within the scope of the preceding text. This includes cardiac tamponade, venous air embolism and fat embolism.

PERICARDIAL TAMPONADE

As a result of misinformation, implanted by textbooks, copied from authority to authority and perpetuated by teachers of physical diagnosis, the diagnosis of pericardial tamponade is generally made late or missed entirely. It is commonly believed, for example, that in pericardial tamponade the neck veins are of necessity distended, the heart sounds muffled, the force of the apex impulse dampened, a friction rub, previously present, decreased in intensity or now absent, orthopnea prominent, the venous pressure elevated, the ventricular pulsations diminished on fluoroscopy and that there must be a characteristic change in the shape of the cardiac silhouette on change in position. While it is true that these signs may be observed in pericardial tamponade they are not invariably present and their absence does not rule out the diagnosis.[1] In 17 patients with proved pericardial tamponade observed by Williams and Soutter [1] the venous pressure was elevated in none judging by examination of the neck veins with the patient seated upright. Much more helpful in this diagnosis was visible pulsation of the neck veins as observed by oblique illumination and the sphygmomanometric detection of a pulsus paradoxus of more than 5 mm. on deep but not maximal inspiration. These signs, to be sure, are not specific, since pulsating veins may be seen in tricuspid regurgitation, pulmonary embolism and constrictive pericarditis and pulsus paradoxus may be observed in any condition associated with pronounced respiratory effort such as bronchial asthma, pneumothorax or congestive heart failure, but their presence may serve as a very useful clue to this diagnosis.

It is noteworthy that in the experimental animal the progressive introduction of fluid into the pericardium induces a very slow rise in venous pressure and fall in systemic arterial pressure until a certain critical level is reached.[2] After this further increments of pericardial fluid of like magnitude and speed produce changes in these parameters much more rapidly. Conversely, with a larger volume of pericardial fluid, the removal of only small amounts may induce profound changes in venous and arterial pressure. This explains the dramatic improvement which may follow the removal of only a few cc. of pericardial fluid (Fig. 43).

It may be worth-while to do a pericardial tap merely to establish the diagnosis; this may be a lead to subsequent emergency therapy. It may help identify the etiologic agent. And finally, and most important, it may prove lifesaving. Just when a tap should be done is extremely difficult to define and is best left to the judgment of the individual physician. A decision is much easier when it is known that there is, rather than that there might be, fluid in the pericardium. A number of techniques have been used; in our experience the safest approach is

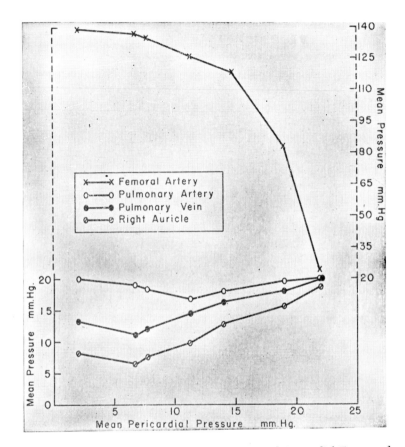

Fig. 43. *Intravascular Pressures in Acute Experimental Pericardial Tamponade.*
As saline is successively infused into the pericardial sac of the dog the systemic
blood pressure (femoral artery x———x) decreases as the venous pressure reflecting right atrial pressure (ø———ø) rises. The curves are gradual with the
earlier accessions in pericardial pressure, abrupt with later additions. Collapse
may therefore occur with small increments on the steep part of the curve. If
the percardium is tapped the fluid may gush out when the pericardial pressure
is high, but may have to be aspirated when the pericardium is under low
pressure. (Reproduced by permission of Evans, J. M., Walter, C. W. and
Hellems, H. K. from data in "Alteration in circulation during cardiac tamponade
due to pericardial effusion. An experimental study employing cardiac catheterization." Am. Ht. J. 39: 181, 1950.)

[355]

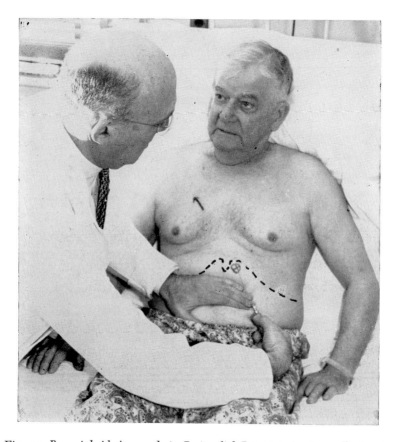

Fig. 44. *Para-xiphoid Approach in Pericardial Paracentesis.* Generally has to be performed with patient in orthopneic position. The needle is introduced just to the left of the xiphoid process and is advanced cephalad, rightward and slightly posteriorly aiming for the right shoulder. To make identification of landmarks easier, preparation of patient and physician are omitted in this figure. *Pericardial tap carries certain hazards and should not be lightly undertaken.*

from just below and to the left of the xiphoid. A blunt, large (e.g. size 16) trochar is maneuvered behind the xiphoid process in a cephalad and posterior direction aiming at the right shoulder so that the pericardium is entered without opening the pleura. The first few centimeters may gush out but the remainder must generally be aspirated. For a number of reasons it is probably preferable to carry out this procedure in the operating room, but this is not always necessary. This subject is further considered on pages 90 and 103.

VENOUS AIR EMBOLISM

This is a potentially fatal but, apparently, reversible emergency. If therapy is to be effective, the diagnosis must be made immediately. The most important ingredient to its recognition is a knowledge of the various circumstances in which it may occur. All of them are iatrogenic and connected with diagnostic or therapeutic procedures which somehow permit the entrance of air into a systemic vein. This includes *surgical operations* (those involving the veins of the neck, thorax or pelvis; direct vision operations on the heart; neurosurgical operations, performed with the patient in the sitting position, and during which the dural sinuses or veins around the cervical or upper thoracic regions of the vertebral column are opened; and uterine curettage with subsequent air insufflation), *diagnostic air injections* (direct or transuterine peritoneal cavity injections; peri-renal air insufflation; injections into the presacral cavity, urinary bladder or large joints; encephalography; or angiography), *therapeutic air injections* (maxillary antrum lavage; pneumoperitoneum; pneumothorax; vaginal powder insufflation, especially during pregnancy; *obstetrical procedures* (during delivery when the patient has a placenta previa; attempted criminal abortion) and from the *accidental entrance of air* (through faulty intravenous apparatus; during phlebotomy;

or from the use of air to speed up transfusion therapy).[3]

The pressure in the right atrium is lower than that in the great veins. And that in the great veins is lower than the pressure in the tributary veins. This pressure gradient explains how air that enters the veins may be floated along the venous stream into the right side of the heart. If enough air enters over a short enough period of time air accumulates in the main pulmonary artery where a frothy "air lock" forms. This obstruction leads in turn to elevated venous pressure, cyanosis, often syncope, deficient cardiac output and a rapid, feeble pulse. Some of the air may pass into the lungs embolizing small and medium-sized pulmonary arteries and producing dyspnea, hyperpnea, and tachypnea.[4] The presence of air in the right ventricle produces a pathognomonic churning sound ("mill-wheel murmur") which may often be heard without a stethoscope, but which can easily be missed in the confusion that frequently exists. The diagnosis may first be made when thoracotomy is performed for cardiac standstill. At this time it is discovered that the right heart is ballooned out and feels like a large bag of air. In an appropriate clinical setting and with a patient who has hitherto done well, the abrupt cessation of respiration and the detection of a "mill-wheel murmur" places the burden of proof on the physician who says that this is not air embolism.

Treatment consists of immediately discontinuing the procedure known to cause, or suspected of causing, the air embolism and immediately having the patient lie on his left side.[5,6,7] By gravity this displaces air from the outflow tract of the right ventricle into the space beneath the tricuspid valve or away from the main pulmonary artery into the radicles of the right pulmonary artery where it is harmless. This preserves the continuity of flow through the right side of the heart. At the same time the patient's head should be kept in a horizontal or dependent position to prevent cerebral embolization. Artificial respiration is indicated if the ordinary reflex stimulation to ventilation is disturbed. The airway should be clear and oxygen administered. There is now a formidable body of evidence documenting the efficacy of this procedure. Should this maneuver prove ineffective and cardiac arrest occur, emergency thoracotomy should be carried out at once, air evacuated from the right side of the heart with syringe and needle followed by cardiac massage. One may spend a moment attempting percutaneous needle aspiration [8] if there is still a heart beat. This is performed while the patient continues to lie in the left lateral position, the needle piercing the fourth intercostal space to the right of the sternum. This should be abandoned immediately if the right ventricle is not entered promptly and thoracotomy should be carried out instead, utilizing ventricular puncture and needle-and-syringe aspiration of air.

FAT EMBOLISM

This is almost certainly a much more common condition than is generally appreciated. It does not produce a distinctive symptomatology. The pathologist does not commonly spur us on to make the correct diagnosis for it is frequently missed as an incidental or primary condition at post-mortem. There may be no suggestion whatever of this condition on gross examination and, with a hasty miscroscopic examination, the non-staining droplets can easily be overlooked in sections stained in the routine manner.[9] A special stain for fat is necessary to establish the diagnosis.

There are three major causes of fat embolism: [10,11,12] (1) *traumatic,* following fractures of the long, marrow-containing bones or orthopedic manipulations particularly of atrophic diseased bone; (2) *metabolic,* the result of an alteration in the physical state of the fats in the blood from a fine to a coarse suspension as in diabetes mellitus, chronic nephritis,

[359]

pancreatitis, chronic tuberculosis, acute and chronic alcoholism, infection with Clostridium perfringens and the injudicious intravenous injection of Vitamin K oxide; and (3) *toxic* as following the ingestion or inhalation of chloroform, ether, carbon monoxide, alcohol, potassium chlorate, phosphorus, carbon tetrachloride or arsenical compounds. Just how these substances induce fat embolism is not known.

The fat thus mobilized may be carried to the lungs, inducing a respiratory symptom complex resembling pneumonia or it may pass on into the systemic circulation embolizing brain, skin, kidneys and other viscera. The symptoms are predominantly cerebral or pulmonary. In the skin fat embolism produces a petechial or purpuric eruption over the neck, shoulders, upper chest or rarely the lower extremities. Ophthalmoscopic examination may also show petechial hemorrhages. The diagnosis is established by the demonstration of fat globules in the sputum or urine using an appropriate fat-staining technique or by the so-called "sizzle" test. A small amount of sputum or urine is put on a platinum loop and the latter then placed in a flame. Normally the water quickly boils away. If fat is present it sizzles and pops in a very characteristic way. Treatment is ill-defined. On the basis of its known effects of clearing the serum of smaller sized fat aggregates, heparin has been suggested as worthy of trial.[13] Until more is known about its value the use of heparin is therefore recommended in the same dose as is used for thromboembolic disease.

REFERENCES

(1) Williams, C. and Soutter, L.: Pericardial tamponade. Diagnosis and treatment. A.M.A. Arch. Int. Med. 94: 571, 1954.
(2) Evans, J. M., Walter, C. W. and Hellems, H. K.: Alterations in the circulation during cardiac tamponade due

to pericardial effusion; an experimental study employing cardiac catheterization. Am. Ht. J. 39: 181, 1950.

(3) Nicholson, M. J.: Emergency treatment of air embolism. In Symposium on Emergency Treatment. Lahey Clinic Bulletin 9: 239. 1956.

(4) Cohen, A. C., Glinsky, G. C., Martin, G. E. and Fetterhoff, K. I.: Air embolism, Ann. Int. Med. 35: 779, 1951.

(5) Durant, T. M., Long, J. and Oppenheimer, M. J.: Pulmonary (venous) air embolism. Am. Ht. J. 33: 269, 1947.

(6) Durant, T. M., Oppenheimer, M. J., Lynch, P. R., Ascanio, G. and Webber, D.: Body position in relation to venous air embolism: a roentgenologic study. Am. J. Med. Sci. 227: 509, 1954.

(7) Musgrove, J. E. and MacQuigg, R. E.: Successful treatment of air embolism. J.A.M.A.: 150: 28, 1952.

(8) Schmidt, P. J. and Kevy, S. V.: Air embolism. A hazard during phlebotomy. N.E.J. Med. 258: 424, 1958.

(9) Swartz, J. H., Tolman, M. M. and Levine, H. D.: Fatality following bismarsen therapy. Arch. Derm. and Syph. 33: 874, 1936.

(10) Warthin, A. S.: Traumatic lipemia and fatty embolism. Internat. Clin. 4: 171, 1913.

(11) Landois, F.: Die Fettembolie. Ergebd. d. Chir. u. Orthop. 16: 99, 1923.

(12) Wright, R. B.: Fat embolism. Ann. Surg. 96: 75, 1932.

(13) Sage, R. H. and Tudor, R. W.: Treatment of fat embolism with heparin. Brit. Med. J. 1: 1160, 1958.

INDEX

INDEX

A

Abdominal cramps
quinidine and, 284
Abdominal paracentesis
congestive heart failure and, 136
digitalis intoxication and, 175
Aberrant ventricular conduction
paroxysmal atrial tachycardia with, 196, 203
quinidine and, 228
Ace binders
thrombophlebitis and, 128
Acute cor pulmonale
chest pain in, 87
electrocardiographic features, 121–123
myocardial infarct simulated by, 123
pulmonary embolism and, 117
right bundle branch block and, 123
Acute coronary insufficiency
acute cor pulmonale and, 118
dissecting aneurysm and, 89
hiatus hernia differentiated from, 107
Acute left ventricular failure
acute myocardial infarction and, 22, 35
acute pulmonary embolism and, 35
alcohol as "anti-foaming" agent in, 32
aminophylline in, 33
aortic embolism precipitating, 34
aortic regurgitation and, 22
aortic stenosis and, 22
Arfonad for, 34
"bloodless phlebotomy" in, 23–25
bronchial asthma, differentiation, 22
carotid sinus stimulation for, 33
coronary artery disease and, 22
Demerol in, 23
digitalis in, 32
ganglionic blocking agents for, 34
hypertensive heart disease and, 22
hypotensive therapy in, 33
morphine in, 22
nitroglycerin for, 33
oxygen therapy in, 29

paroxysmal rapid heart action and, 35
phlebotomy in, 26
pulmonary infarction and, 117
renal infarction precipitating, 34
salt infusion and, 147
venous tourniquets in, 23–25
mitral stenosis and, 21, 22
Serpasil for, 34
tourniquet in, 17
Acute mediastinal emphysema, 93–97
chest pain in, 87
rupture of esophagus and, 99
Acute myocardial infarction
acute cor pulmonale simulating, 123
acute left ventricular failure and, 22, 35
acute mediastinal emphysema differentiated from, 94
acute pericarditis differentiated from, 102
anticoagulant therapy in, 17, 68–78
"arm chair" treatment for, 67
atrial fibrillation during, 257
cardiac resuscitation during, 347, 348
chest wall syndrome and, 105
complete heart block in, 296
dicumarol in, 70–74
dissecting aneurysm of aorta with, 89, 90
dihydromorphinone hydrochloride for, 63
extension of infarct in, 62
Heparin for, 69, 74
hiatus hernia differentiated from, 107
hypotension in, 41
lipo-hepin in, 69
morphine in, 62
nitroglycerin in, 67
oxygen for, 66
paroxysmal atrial tachycardia simulating, 192
paroxysmal ventricular tachycardia and, 263
pulmonary embolism misdiagnosed as, 116

"refractory" congestive failure and, 135
shock in, 39, 40
syncope and, 324
Acute pericarditis, 102–104
Acute pulmonary edema,
(see acute left ventricular failure)
Acute pulmonary embolism
acute left ventricular failure precipitated by, 35
anticoagulant therapy in, 125, 126
caval ligation and, 127
common femoral vein ligation and, 126
elastic stockings and, 127
"refractory" congestive failure and, 135
shock in, 39, 47
thrombophlebitis and, 124–128
Acute rheumatic carditis
complete heart block in, 296
"refractory" congestive failure and, 135
Adams-Stokes Disease
(see complete heart block)
Addisonian crisis
potassium intoxication in, 156
Adrenal insufficiency
shock and, 44
Adrenalin
(see epinephrine)
Agranulocytosis
phenindione producing, 75
Air embolism, venous
causes of, 357
"Air lock"
venous air embolism and, 358
Alcohol
angina pectoris and, 57
"anti-foaming" effect of, 37
atrial fibrillation and, 256
Alcoholism
rupture of esophagus and, 99
Aldactone
aldosterone-inhibiting effect of, 149
Alkali therapy
hiatus hernia and, 107, 108
Allen's sign
pulmonary embolism and, 117
Alternation in cycle length
paroxysmal atrial tachycardia and, 196
paroxysmal ventricular tachycardia with, 265, 266

Aminophylline
acute ventricular failure and, 33
"merc-sandwich" diuresis with, 149
Ammonium chloride
congestive failure treated with, 145, 146
hypochloremic alkalosis treated with, 143, 144
Ammonium intoxication, 144–146
"cardiac psychosis" and, 135
digitalis intoxication and, 175, 178
Amyl nitrite
angina pectoris and, 56
Anemia, 26, 135
Aneurysm of aorta, syphilitic
chest pain in, 87
Angina pectoris
acute cor pulmonale and, 118
acute mediastinal emphysema differentiation from, 94
alcohol for, 57
amyl nitrite for, 56
aortic valve disease and, 57
blood pressure during, 53
carotid sinus stimulation, 54, 57
clinical features, 53
deep inspiration and, 54
electrocardiogram during, 54
erythrol tetranitrate for, 57
hemorrhage and, 57
hypoglycemia and, 56
nerve root pain differentiated from, 97
nitroglycerin in, 54–57
octyl nitrite for, 56
paroxysmal atrial tachycardia and, 59
paroxysmal rapid heart action and, 57
subendocardial ischemia in, 54
thyrotoxicosis and, 57
Anoxic syncope, 325
Ansolysen
coronary insufficiency precipitated by, 61
Anterior chest wall syndrome, 105
Anorexia
digitalis induced, 176, 177
Anticoagulant therapy
acute myocardial infarction and, 17, 68–78
acute pulmonary embolism and, 125, 126

INDEX

atrial fibrillation and, 258
blood dyscrasias and, 68
contraindication to, 68
coumadin in, 75, 76
cyclocumerol in, 75
diphenedione in, 75
ethyl biscoumacetate in, 75
hematuria and, 68
hemopericardium complicating, 76
hemorrhage in, 76
liver disease and, 68
melena and, 68
peptic ulcer and, 68, 76
phenindione in, 75
tamponade complicating, 76
uterine bleeding and, 77
Aortic embolism
acute left ventricular failure precipitated by, 34
Aortic regurgitation
acute left ventricular failure in, 22
dissecting aneurysm of aorta and,
90
Aortic stenosis
acute left ventricular failure in, 22
syncope and, 324
Aortic valve disease
angina pectoris and, 57
Apomorphine, 205
Aphonia, 165
Aramine
(see metaraminol)
Areolae, hyperpigmentation of, 179
Arfonad, 34, 326
Arginine, 145
"Arm chair" treatment
acute myocardial infarction and, 67
congestive heart failure and, 137–
141
Arrhythmias
"refractory" congestive failure and,
135
shock induced by, 47
Arterial thrombosis
thrombolytic agents in, 78
Arthritis of spine
chest pain from, 87
Artificial kidney, 162
Artificial respiration, 338
"Ashman phenomenon"
aberrant ventricular conduction
and, 180
Asthma

acute mediastinal emphesema in,
93
Atabrine
paroxysmal atrial tachycardia and,
208
Atrial fibrillation
acute myocardial infarction complicated by, 257
alcohol and, 256
anticoagulant therapy for, 258
atrial flutter differentiated from,
223, 253
atrial premature beats differentiated
from, 252
atrial tachycardia with block differentiated from, 238, 253
clinical features, 249–252
complete heart block with, 252
cortisone in, 258
digitalis in treatment of, 255
digitalis intoxication and, 252
embolism complicating, 250
mitral valvuloplasty and, 257, 258
nodal tachycardia with, 184, 252
Ouabain in treatment of, 256
paroxysmal ventricular tachycardia
differentiated from, 253, 254,
273
quinidine, 257, 259
rheumatic carditis and, 258
without heart disease, 256
prostigmine and, intraoperative, 257
shock with, 47
Wolff-Parkinson-White syndrome
and, 193
Atrial flutter
atrial fibrillation differentiated from,
223, 253
atrial tachycardia with block differentiation from, 238–240
carotid sinus stimulation and, 202,
219
clinical features, 220–223
digitalis in treatment of, 226
electrocardiographic features, 215–
219
first sound and, 201
lability of heart rate in, 220
1:1 response in
paroxysmal atrial tachycardia differentiated from, 201
paroxysmal ventricular tachycardia
differentiated from, 273

[367]

quinidine and, 227–230
quinidine inducing, 282
shock with, 47
with intraventricular block
    paroxysmal ventricular tachycardia differentiated from, 224, 225
Wolff-Parkinson-White syndrome and, 193
Atrial premature beats
    atrial fibrillation differentiated from, 252
    digitalis intoxication and, 183
Atrial sounds
    complete heart block, 298
Atrial standstill, 160
Atrial tachycardia with block
    atrial fibrillation differentiated from, 238, 253
    atrial flutter differentiated from, 238–240
    atrial rhythm in, 236
    (digitalis induced)
        potassium in treatment of, 242–244
    digitalis intoxication and, 240
    electrocardiographic features, 236
    "latent" block in, 236
    Na-EDTA in treatment of, 244
    (non-digitalis induced)
        digitalis in treatment of, 242
    P wave in, 236
    paroxysmal atrial tachycardia differentiated from, 202
    paroxysmal ventricular tachycardia differentiated from, 273, 274
    procaine amide in treatment of, 244
Atrioventricular block
    atrioventricular dissociation distinguished from, 184
    potassium depletion and, 168
    potassium intoxication and, 158
Atrioventricular block complete
    (see complete heart block)
Atrioventricular dissociation, 184
    digitalis intoxication and, 184
    paroxysmal ventricular tachycardia and, 265, 266
Atropine, 125, 279, 280, 303, 316, 319, 323
Autonomic nervous system, 318

Azygos vein, dilatation of
    acute cor pulmonale and, 121

B

Bacterial endocarditis, subacute
    (see subacute bacterial endocarditis)
Ball valve thrombus, 324
Barbiturates
    "cardiac psychosis" and, 135
Bedpan "blackouts"
    Valsalva maneuver and, 322
Belladonna, 107, 108, 303, 316
Bicarbonate concentration, serum, 142
Bidirectional ventricular tachycardia
    digitalis intoxication and, 276, 285
Bigeminal rhythm, 182, 183
Blast injuries, 94
Blindness, 89
Blood dyscrasias, 68
Blood pressure
    dissecting aneurysm of aorta and, 88
Blood pressure level
    phlebotomy and, 26
"Bloodless phlebotomy," 23, 25
Blow to pericardium
    ventricular standstill and, 305
    cardiac resuscitation and, 338, 340
Bradycardia
    cardiac arrest heralded by, 335
    potassium intoxication and, 156
Bronchial asthma, 22
Bronchopneumonia
    pulmonary embolism and, 116
"Bruit de canon"
    complete heart block and, 298
Bundle branch block, 160
Bundle branch block partial (2:1), 278

C

Caisson disease, 94
Calcium chloride, 338, 339, 344
Calcium gluconate, 207
Calcium salts, 161
Carbon tetrachloride poisoning, 156
Carcinoma of esophagus, 108
Carcinoma of lung, 87
Cardiac arrest
    digitalis and, 333
    external "pacemaker" and, 340

impending, 334–336
management of, 338–345
manual systole for, 339, 340, 342
potassium intoxication and, 155, 161
predisposing conditions, 333, 334
quinidine and, 333
recognition of, 337, 338
Cardiac output
bigeminal rhythm and, 183
"Cardiac psychosis"
heart disease and, 135
digitalis intoxication and, 178
Cardiac silhouette
pericardial tamponade and, 353
Cardiac surgery
ventricular standstill and, 334
Cardiac work
"arm-chair" treatment and, 137
"Cardiogenic shock"
(see shock)
Carotid sinus sensitivity
atropine for, 316
detection of, 315, 316
ephedrine for, 316
functional hypoglycemia and, 316, 328
tight collar and, 317
Carotid sinus stimulation
acute left ventricular failure and, 33
atrial flutter and, 219
cerebral thrombosis induced by, 315
complete heart block induced by, 292
paroxysmal atrial tachycardia and, 194, 201, 204, 205
paroxysmal ventricular tachycardia and, 265, 269, 273
Carotid sinus stimulation test
angina pectoris and, 54, 57
Carotid sinus syncope, 314–317
Caval ligation, 127
Cedilanid, 206
Cerebral thrombosis
carotid sinus stimulation and, 205, 315
Chelating agents, 187
Chest deformities, 23
Chest pain
acute mediastinal emphysema and, 93, 94

causes, 87
dissecting aneurysm in, 87, 88
paroxysmal ventricular tachycardia and, 265, 279
Chest trauma, 94
Chlorothiazide, 146, 148, 175, 318
Cholelithiasis, 296
Chronic constrictive pericarditis, 104
"refractory" congestive failure and, 135
Cinchonism, 284
Cirrhosis of the liver
ammonium intoxication and, 144
Clotting time, 69
Coarctation of the aorta
dissection of aorta complicating, 88
Collapse
nitroglycerin as cause, 55
Colored vision, 177, 178
Coma
potassium intoxication and, 158
Common femoral vein ligation, 126
Common carotid artery, left, 89
Compazine
(see prochlorperazine)
Complete heart block
acute myocardial infarction and, 296
atrial fibrillation with, 252
atrial sounds in, 298
"bruit de canon" in, 298
carotid sinus stimulation inducing, 292
congenital heart disease and, 296
coronary artery disease and, 296
cortisone for, 304
digitalis in treatment of, 300
ephedrine in, 303
epinephrine and, 299, 300
first sound in, 297, 298
hypertensive heart disease and, 296
isopropyl-arterenol and, 299, 303, 305, 307
"pacemaker" in, 301
paroxysmal ventricular tachycardia and, 264, 292
sodium lactate in, 303
sympathico-mimetic amines and, 299, 300
ventricular fibrillation and, 292, 293
ventricular standstill in, 292

ventricular rate in, 296
Congenital heart disease, 325
Congestive heart failure
abdominal paracentesis in, 136
ammonium intoxication in, 144–146
"arm-chair" treatment, 137–141
atrial tachycardia with block and, 235
digitalis intoxication and, 174, 175
paroxysmal ventricular tachycardia precipitating, 279
phlebotomy in, 46, 136
pulmonary embolism and, 117, 118
shock in, 39, 47
Southey's tubes and, 136
syncope and, 322
thoracentesis in, 136
Constrictive pericarditis
(see chronic constrictive pericarditis)
Contour pillow, 99
Convulsions, 118
Cor pulmonale, acute
(see acute cor pulmonale)
Coronary artery disease
acute left ventricular failure in, 22
chest wall syndrome and, 105
complete heart block and, 296
intravenous therapy in, 65
paroxysmal atrial tachycardia and, 193
paroxysmal ventricular tachycardia and, 263
Coronary artery disease, pain in, 97
Coronary insufficiency
"Coronary regimen" for, 59
heparin for, 60
hypotensive therapy as cause, 61
meperidine for, 59
morphine for, 59
nitroglycerin for, 59
symptomatology, 58
Coronary nodal rhythm
paroxysmal atrial tachycardia and, 193
Cortisone, 44, 258, 304
Costochondral syndrome
(see Tietze's syndrome)
Coumadin, 75, 76
Coumarin compounds
prothrombin time, Vitamin K_1 oxide and, 69
Coupled rhythm

digitalis intoxication and, 182, 183
Cumopyron
(see cyclocumarol)
Cupped-depressed RS-T segment
digitalis and, 176
Cyanosis, 31
Cyclocumarol, 75

D

Danilone
(see phenindione)
Deafness
quinidine and, 228, 284
Defibrillator, external, 346, 347
Defibrillator, internal, 339, 345
Delirium, 178
Demerol
(see meperidine)
Denervation of carotid sinus, 317
Desoxycorticosterone, 165, 319
Dextran, 40
Dextrose solution, 344
Diabetic acidosis, 156
Diabetic coma, impending, 87
Diabetic neuropathy, 318
Dialysis, transperitoneal, 163
Diamox, 148, 175
Diarrhoea
dicumarol and, 74
digitalis induced, 176
potassium depletion and, 165
quinidine and, 284
Dicumarol, 70–74
Digitalis
acute left ventricular failure and, 32
atrial fibrillation treated with, 255
atrial flutter and, 226
atrial tachycardia with block (non digitalis induced) treated with, 242
cardiac arrest and, 333
complete heart block treated with, 300
malabsorption of, 141
paroxysmal atrial tachycardia treated with, 206
paroxysmal ventricular tachycardia and, 263
shock and, 46
thyrotoxic heart disease treated with, 256

vasopressor amides potentiated by, 46
Digitalis effect
electrocardiogram, 176
Digitalis glycoside
purified digitalis toxicity and, 174, 176, 177
Digitalis intoxication
alternating bidirectional ventricular tachycardia and, 276
atrial fibrillation and, 252
atrial tachycardia with block and, 240
"cardiac psychosis" and, 135
complete heart block and, 296
paroxysmal ventricular tachycardia and, 276, 285
Digitalization, intravenous, 255
Digitalization, oral, 226
Digitoxin, 186
Digoxin, 186, 206
Dihydromorphinone hydrochloride, 63
Dilaudid
(see didroxymorphinone hydrochloride)
Dipaxin
(see diphenedione)
Diphenedione, 75
Diphtheria
acute mediastinal emphysema from, 93
complete heart block and, 296
Disc, intervertebral, rupture of chest pain and, 97
Dissecting aneurysm of aorta
clinical features, 87–90
hemothorax, left, in, 91
hypertension and, 80
Logue's sign in, 88
roentgen ray in, 91
shock in, 47
surgery for, 91, 92
tamponade in, 90, 91
treatment of, 91, 92
Diuretic agents
digitalis intoxication and, 175
Diuretic therapy
"merc-sandwich" and, 149
renal enzymes and, 148
Diuril
(see chlorthiazide)

coronary insufficiency precipitated by, 61
Dizziness, 118, 284

E

Ectopic rhythm, 43, 299, 300
Edema of legs
vein ligation and, 126
Electrocardiogram
acute cor pulmonale and, 121–123
acute pericarditis and, 102
angina pectoris and, 54
atrial tachycardia with block and, 236
atrial flutter and, 215–219
complete heart block and, digitalis effect, 176
potassium depletion and, 166
potassium intoxication and, 158–160
Electrocardiographic monitoring
potassium intoxication and, 164
Electroencephalogram
ammonium chloride intoxication and, 145
Embolism
anticoagulant therapy for, 258
mitral valvuloplasty for, 258
Emetine
orthostatic hypotension and, 318
Emphysema, subcutaneous
acute mediastinal emphysema and, 95
Ephedrine, 45, 303, 316, 323
Epigastric pain, 74
Epilepsy
syncope due to, 327
Epinephrine
complete heart block and, 299, 300
shock and, 45, 46
ventricular standstill and, 338, 339, 343, 344
in oil
complete heart block and, 299
inhalation
complete heart block and, 303
Erythrol tetranitrite, 57
Esophageal spasm, 57
Esophageal stricture
hiatus hernia and, 107
Ethyl biscoumacetate, 75
Exchange resins
potassium intoxication, treatment with, 162

Exercise
atrial flutter and, 221, 222
External defibrillator, 305, 346, 347
External "pacemaker", 301, 302, 303, 305

F

Faint, simple, 314
Faintness
acute cor pulmonale and, 118
Fainting
dissecting aneurysm of aorta and, 89
Fat embolism, 360
"Fibrillo-flutter", 224
First sound
atrial flutter and, 201, 222
complete heart block and, 297, 298
paroxysmal atrial tachycardia and, 194, 201
paroxysmal ventricular tachycardia and, 265
Fistula, gastrointestinal
potassium depletion and, 165
Flap, hepatic
ammonium intoxication and, 144
Fluorohydrocortisone, 9-alpha
orthostatic hypotension and, 319
Flutter waves in neck
atrial flutter and, 222, 223
"Flutter-fibrillation," 224
Fractures
fat embolism and, 359
Fracture, vertebral
chest pain and, 97
Fractured ribs
acute mediastinal emphysema from, 94
Friction rub
acute pericarditis and, 102
pulmonary infarction and, 118
Fusion ventricular beats
paroxysmal ventricular tachycardia and, 271

G

Gallbladder disease
nitroglycerin and, 51
Ganglionic blocking agents, 34, 318
Gardener's syncope, 328
Glossopharyngeal nerve, section of
carotid sinus sensitivity and, 317
Glucose and insulin, 161

Glutamate, 145
Gumma
complete heart block and, 296
Graft surgery
dissecting aneurysm of aorta and, 91, 92
Green vision, 177, 178

H

Hamman's disease
(see acute mediastinal emphysema)
Hammock-shaped RS-T segment
digitalis and, 176
Headache
nitroglycerin and, 55
Heart sounds, muffled,
pericardial tamponade and, 353
Hedulin
(see phenindione)
Hematocrit level
phlebotomy and, 26
Hematuria
anticoagulant therapy and, 68
Hemodialysis, artificial
potassium intoxication treated with, 162
Hemolytic crises
potassium intoxication and, 156
Hemopericardium
anticoagulant therapy and, 76
chronic constrictive pericarditis and, 104
dissecting aneurysm of aorta and, 90, 91
Hemorrhage, 39, 47, 51, 76, 320
Hemothorax, left
dissecting aneurysm of aorta and, 91
Heparin
acute myocardial infarction and, 69, 74
clotting time and, 69
coronary insufficiency and, 60
dicumarol therapy, 74
fat embolism and, 360
protamine and, 69, 70
Swedish technique, 69
"Hepatic flap"
ammonium intoxication and, 144
Herpes zoster
chest pain and, 87, 97
Hiatus hernia, 106, 107
chest pain and, 87

Hoarseness
  potassium depletion and, 165
Homans' sign
  thrombophlebitis and, 124
Hydrochloric acid, 143
Hydrochlorothiazide, 146, 148
Hydrocortisone derivatives, 149
Hydrodiuril
  (see hydrochlorothiazide)
Hyperaldosteronism
  potassium depletion in, 165
Hypertension
  phlebotomy and, 26
Hypertensive heart disease
  acute left ventricular failure in, 22
  paroxysmal atrial tachycardia and,
    193
Hyperchloremic acidosis, 144–146
Hypertensive encephalopathy
  syncope in, 326
Hypertensive heart disease
  complete heart block and, 296
Hyperventilation syncope
  clinical features of, 317
Hyperventilation syndrome
  hypoglycemia and, 328
Hypochloremic acidosis
  "refractory" congestive failure and,
    142–144
Hypoglycemia
  angina pectoris and, 56
  functional, carotid sinus sensitivity
    and, 316, 328
  functional, hyperventilation syn-
    drome and, 328
Hypoprothrombinemia
  dicumarol and, 70
Hypotension, 41, 335
Hypotensive therapy, 61, 334
Hypothermia
  ventricular standstill and, 334
Hyponatremia
  chlorthiazide as cause, 146
Hypotension
  quinidine and, 228
Hypotensive therapy, 33
Hypoxia
  oxygen therapy for, 31

I

Ileus
  potassium depletion and, 165
Inanedione compounds

  prothrombin time and, 69
  Vitamin K_1 oxide and, 69
Infarction, myocardial
  (see acute myocardial infarction)
Infarction, pulmonary
  (see pulmonary infarction)
Infection
  shock in, 39
Innominate artery, compression
  dissecting aneurysm of aorta and,
    87
Inspiration
  angina pectoris relieved by, 54
Insulin, 161, 165
Intestinal intubation
  potassium depletion and, 165
Intra-atrial block, 158, 282
Intracranial surgery
  ventricular standstill and, 334
Intratracheal insufflation
  acute mediastinal emphysema and,
    93
Intraventricular block
  paroxysmal atrial tachycardia with,
    196, 203
  potassium intoxication and, 160
  procaine amide and, 282
  quinidine and, 228
  quinidine toxicity and, 282
Ipecac
  paroxysmal atrial tachycardia
    treated with, 205
Isopropyl-arterenol
  complete heart block and, 299, 303,
    305, 307

J

Jaundice
  pulmonary infarction and, 118
Jugular pulse
  paroxysmal ventricular tachycardia
    and, 265

K

Kay-exalate
  potassium intoxication treated with,
    162
Kidney disease
  digitalis intoxication and, 174
  unilateral, orthostatic hypotension
    and, 319
Knee-chest position
  hypoxia relieved by, 325

L

Lactic acid dehydrogenese, serum
 pulmonary infarction and, 120
Laryngeal obstruction
 acute mediastinal emphysema from,
 93
Lassitude
 dicumarol and, 72
 quinidine and, 284
Left lateral decubitus
 air embolism and, 358
Left ventricular failure
 (see acute left ventricular failure)
Levophed
 (see nor-epinephrine)
Lipo-hepin
 acute myocardial infarction and, 69
Liver disease
 anticoagulant therapy and, 68
 digitalis intoxication and, 174
Logue's sign
 dissecting aneurysm of aorta and,
 88
Low sodium syndrome
 salt restriction and, 146

M

Magnesium sulfate, 208, 284
Manual systole
 ventricular fibrillation and, 339,
 345, 346
 ventricular standstill and, 339, 340
Mecholyl
 paroxysmal atrial tachycardia and,
 206
Mediastinal emphysema, acute
 (see acute mediastinal emphysema)
Melena, 68
Meperidine, 23, 59, 63
Mephentermine, 41, 42, 45, 207
Mephyton
 (see Vitamin K_1 oxide)
Mercurial diuresis
 digitalis intoxication and, 175
 low sodium syndrome and, 146
 potassium depletion and, 165
Mesenteric embolism
 shock in, 47
Mesenteric thrombosis
 dissecting aneurysm of aorta in, 89
Metaraminol
 shock and, 41, 45

Methoxamine, 41, 42, 45, 207
Methyl prednisolone, 149
Micturition syncope
 nitroglycerin in, 56
 Valsalva maneuver and, 322
"Mill-wheel murmur"
 venous air embolism and, 358
"Mitral" P waves
 quinidine effect simulating, 282
Mitral stenosis, 21, 22, 135
Mitral valvuloplasty
 atrial fibrillation and, 257
 embolism and, 258
Morphine
 acute left ventricular failure and, 22
 acute myocardial infarction and, 62
 acute pulmonary embolism and, 125
 chest deformities, 23
 coronary insufficiency and, 59
 orthostatic hypotension and, 318
 pulmono-cardiac failure and, 23
 shock and, 46
Mouth-to-mouth breathing, 338
Multiple sclerosis
 orthostatic hypotension and, 318
Myocardial infarction, acute
 (see acute myocardial infarction)
Myxoma of atrium
 syncope and, 325

N

Nasal catheter, 29
Nasogastric suction
 potassium depletion and, 165
Nausea
 digitalis induced, 176
 quinidine and, 284
Neck veins, distension of
 pericardial tamponade and, 353
 pulsation of, pericardial tamponade
 and, 354
Necrosis of tissue
 nor-epinephrine and, 43
Needle stimulation of heart
 cardiac resuscitation and, 338, 340
 ventricular standstill and, 305
Neohydrin
 tandem diuretic therapy including,
 148
Neomycin, 145
Neosynephrine
 (see phenylephrine hydrochloride)
Nerve root pain, 97–99

Nitroglycerin
acute left ventricular failure and, 33
acute myocardial infarction and, 67
angina pectoris and, 54–57
collapse from, 55
coronary insufficiency and, 59
esophageal spasm relieved by, 59
gallbladder disease and, 57
headache from, 55
orthostatic hypertension and, 318
Nodal tachycardia
atrial fibrillation with, 184, 252
digitalis intoxication and, 184
Nor-epinephrine, 41, 43, 44, 207

O

Obstetrical procedure
venous air embolism and, 357
Octyl nitrite, 56
Ocular pressure, 205
Oligemic syncope, 320, 321
Orange vision, 177, 178
Oro-pharyngeal tube, 338
Orthostatic hypotension, 318
Ouabain, 186, 256
Oxygen therapy
acute left ventricular failure and, 29
acute mediastinal emphysema and, 97
acute myocardial infarction and, 66
acute pulmonary embolism and, 125
alcohol as "anti-foaming" agent in, 32
cyanosis and, 31
face mask technique, 30
nasal catheter technique, 29
oxygen tent for, 29, 31

P

P wave
paroxysmal atrial tachycardia and, 196
"Pacemaker"
application of, 301
complete heart block and, 301
external cardiac arrest and, 340, 346
ventricular standstill and, 339
Packed red cells
transfusion of, 29
Pancreatitis, acute, 87

Paracentesis
potassium depletion and, 165
Paracentesis, pericardial
acute pericarditis and, 103
Paraplegia
dissecting aneurysm of aorta and, 89
Parkinson-Papp syndrome, 196
Paroxysmal atrial tachycardia, 191–193, 202, 273
Paroxysmal nodal tachycardia, 273, 276
with intraventricular block, 269, 270
Paroxysmal rapid heart action
acute left ventricular failure and, 35
angina pectoris and, 57
Paroxysmal ventricular tachycardia
atrial fibrillation differentiated from, 253, 254
atrial flutter with intraventricular block differentiated from, 224, 225
clinical features, 264, 265
complete heart block and, 292
digitalis intoxication and, 185
electrocardiographic features, 268–271
external defibrillator for, 305
potassium intoxication and, 160
procaine amide inducing, 282
quinidine and, 228, 282
shock in, 47
Parturition
acute mediastinal emphysema and, 93
Peaked T waves
potassium intoxication and, 158
Pericardial paracentesis
hemopericardium and, 77
pericardial tamponade and, 354–357
Pericardial tamponade, 354–357
Pericarditis, acute, 87
Periodic paralysis, 165
Peptic esophagitis, 107, 108
Peptic ulcer, 68, 76, 87
Percussion of spine
nerve root pain and, 97
Pertussis
acute mediastinal emphysema from, 93

Petechiae
  fat embolism and, 359
Pheninedione, 75
Phentolamine, 43, 44
Phenylephrine hydrochloride, 41, 42, 45, 207
Pheochromocytoma
  orthostatic hypotension and, 319
Phlebothrombosis
  (see thrombophlebitis)
Phlebotomy
  acute left ventricular failure and, 26
  congestive heart failure and, 136
  congestive heart failure and shock treated with, 46
  hematocrit level and, 26
  technique of, 26
Photofluorometric method
  serum quinidine level determined by, 229
Phytonedione
  (see Viatmin K_1 oxide)
Plasma-expanders
  shock and, 40
Pleural effusion
  rupture of esophagus and, 99
  hemorrhagic pulmonary infarction and, 118
Pleurisy, acute
  chest pain in, 87
Pneumonia
  chest pain in, 87
Pneumopericardium
  acute mediastinal emphysema and, 94
Pneumothorax
  (see spontaneous pneumothorax)
  tension type, acute mediastinal emphysema complicated by, 96
Polyethylene catheter
  nor-epinephrine and, 43
Popping sound
  acute mediastinal emphysema, and 95
Postural strain
  chest pain and, 97
Posture
  hiatus hernia and, 106
  pericarditis and, 102
  "pericardial catch" and, 105
  syncope and, 313
  Tietze's syndrome and, 104

Potassium
  atrial tachycardia with block (digitalis induced) treated with, 242–244
  ventricular fibrillation treated with, 346
Potassium depletion
  cardiac arrest and, 333
  chlorothiazid as cause, 146
  clinical features, 164–166
  digitalis intoxication and, 175
  electrocardiographic features, 166–168
  low sodium syndrome and, 148
Potassium intoxication
  cardiac arrest and, 333
  paroxysmal ventricular tachycardia in, 264, 284
"Potassium-losing" nephritis
  potassium depletion in, 165
Potassium therapy, 186
"Precordial catch", 105
Prednisolone, 149
Pregnancy, 88, 320
Premature beats, atrial
  (see atrial premature beats)
Premature beats, ventricular
  (see ventricular premature beats)
Prochlorperazine, 22
Procaine amide
  atrial tachycardia with block treated with, 244
  cardiac arrest and, 333
  complete heart block and, 304
  digitalis intoxication and, 186
  intraventricular block and, 282
  paroxysmal ventricular tachycardia due to, 263, 264
  paroxysmal ventricular tachycardia treated with, 278, 280
  toxicity of, 281–284
Procaine injection, 98
Propatheline bromide, 107, 108
Prostigmine, 206
Protamine
  heparin and, 69, 70
Prothrombin time
  coumarin compounds and, 69
  optimal
    "escape" from, 72
Psychogenic syncope, 314
Pulmonary atelectasis
  pulmonary infarction and, 121

Pulmonary edema acute
(see acute left ventricular failure)
Pulmonary embolism
(see acute pulmonary embolism)
Pulmonary infarction
chest pain in, 87
clinical syndrome, 116
physical findings in, 118, 119
pulmonary atelectasis and, 121
Pulmonic second sound
acute cor pulmonale and, 119
Pulsating mass, abdominal
dissecting aneurysm of aorta and,
89
"Pulse deficit"
atrial fibrillation and, 250
Pulses, radial
dissecting aneurysm of aorta and,
89
Pulsus paradoxus
pericardial tamponade and, 354
"Pyramiding" effect
quinidine and, 229

Q

Q-T interval
digitalis and, 176
potassium depletion and, 166
Quinacrine hydrochloride, 208
Quinidine
atrial fibrillation treated with, 257,
259
atrial flutter and, 227–230
cardiac arrest from, 333
complete heart block and, 304
orthostatic hypotension and, 318
Paroxysmal atrial tachycardia treated
with, 206
paroxysmal ventricular tachycardia
due to, 263, 264
treated with, 278–284
toxicity of, 228
ventricular acceleration and, 228
Quinidine toxicity
intraventricular block and, 282
Quinidinization, intravenous
technique for, 279, 280
oral
technique for, 227
Quinine, 280

R

RS-T segment

digitalis effect upon, 176
depression of
potassium depletion and, 166
Rauwolfia preparations, 61, 318
Re-expansion of lungs
spontaneous pneumothorax and,
108, 109
Refractory period
aberrant ventricular conduction and,
180
"Refractory" congestive heart failure,
148, 149
Regitine
(see phentolamine)
"Regular irregularity"
atrial flutter and, 217, 223
Renal infarction
acute left ventricular failure precipitated by, 34
Repetitive paroxysmal atrial tachycardia
rhythm in, 196
Reserpine, 326
Respiratory arrest, 284
Retinal detachment
ocular pressure and, 205
Retropneumoperitoneum
acute mediastinal emphysema and,
94
Reversible heart disease
"refractoriness" to therapy and,
134, 135
Rheumatic carditis
atrial fibrillation in, 258
cortisone in, 258
Rheumatic heart disease
complete heart block and, 296
paroxysmal atrial tachycardia and,
193
paroxysmal ventricular tachycardia
and, 263
Right bundle branch block
acute cor pulmonale and, 123
Right ventricular failure
responsiveness to therapy in, 133
Roentgen-ray examination
acute cor pulmonale and, 121
acute mediastinal emphysema and,
96
acute pericarditis and, 103
dissecting aneurysm of aorta and,
91
nerve root pain and, 98

pulmonary infarction and, 120
rupture of esophagus and, 100
spontaneous pneumothorax and, 108
Roentgen-ray therapy
Tietze's syndrome and, 105
Root sleeve fibrosis
chest pain and, 97
Rotating tourniquet
acute left ventricular failure and,
25
Rupture of esophagus, 99, 100
acute mediastinal emphysema from,
94
chest pain and, 87
Ruptured intervertebral disc
chest pain and, 97

S

Salicylate, 258
Salt
orthostatic hypotension treated
with, 319
"Salt losing" nephritis
low sodium syndrome and, 147
Salt restriction
digitalis intoxication and, 175
low sodium syndrome and, 146
Second sound, pulmonic
acute cor pulmonale and, 119
Sensitivity to digitalis, 178, 179
Serpasil, 34
Serum quinidine level
photofluorometric determination,
229
Shock
acute pulmonary embolism and, 39,
47
adrenal insufficiency in, 44
arrhythmia as cause, 47
congestive heart failure with, 46,
47
cortisone in, 44
digitalis in, 46
ephedrine in, 45
epinephrine in, 45, 46
hemorrhage and, 47
"irreversible phase" in, 42
isopropyl arterenol and, 46
mephentermine in, 41, 42, 45
mesenteric embolism and, 47
metaraminol in, 41, 45
morphine in, 40
myocardial infarction and, 39

nor-epinephrine in, 41, 42, 43, 44
paroxysmal ventricular tachycardia
and, 47, 279, 285
phenylephrine hydrochloride in, 41,
42, 45
plasma-expanders in, 40
pulmonary infarction and, 117
syncope in, 320
transfusion in, 40
vaso-pressor amines in, 40–46
Shoulder brace, 99
Side-rails
complete heart block and, 298
Sino-atrial block
syncope due to, 323
Sinus tachycardia
digitalis and, 175, 176
paroxysmal atrial tachycardia differentiated from, 200
"Sizzle" test
fat embolism and, 359
Sodium bicarbonate, hypertonic
potassium intoxication treated with,
161
Sodium chloride, hypertonic, 147
Sodium concentration, serum, normal
value, 142
Sodium indiscretion
"refractory" congestive failure and,
135
Sodium lactate
complete heart block treated with,
303
potassium intoxication treated with,
161
Sorbitol
potassium intoxication treated with,
162
Southey's tube
congestive heart failure and, 136
digitalis intoxication and, 175
Spine, percussion of
nerve root pain and, 98
Spinal traction
nerve root pain treated by, 98
Spiro-lactone, 149
Spontaneous pneumothorax
acute mediastinal emphysema and,
94
chest pain in, 87
clinical features, 108
re-expansion of lungs in, 108, 109
roentgen-ray examination in, 108

Sputum, fat, 360
Squatting position
hypoxia relieved by, 325
"Staircase ascent"
acute cor pulmonale and, 123
Sternoclavicular joint, pulsation of
dissecting aneurysm of aorta and,
88
Steroid therapy
ammonium chloride intoxication
treated with, 145
anterior chest wall syndrome and,
105
digitalis intoxication evoked by,
175
diuretic effect, 149
ventricular standstill and, 334
Strain, postural
chest pain and, 97
Streptodornase
thrombolytic effect of, 78
Streptokinase
thrombolytic effect of, 78
Stricture of esophagus
hiatus hernia and, 107
Subacute bacterial endocarditis
as emergency, 15
"refractory" congestive failure and,
135
Subaortic stenosis, congenital
syncope in, 325
Subcutaneous emphysema
acute mediastinal emphysema and,
95
rupture of esophagus and, 99
Subendocardial ischemia
angina pectoris and, 54
Subluxation, vertebral
chest pain and, 97
Supraclavicular incision
acute emphysema treated by, 96
Surgery
hiatus hernia and, 107, 108
venous air embolism and, 357
Sympathectomy
orthostatic hypotension and, 318
paroxysmal ventricular tachycardia
treated with, 285
Sympathico-mimetic amines, 40–46
complete heart block and, 299, 300
Syncope
acute cor pulmonale and, 118
aortic stenosis and, 324

benign, 314
paroxysmal atrial tachycardia and,
192
paroxysmal ventricular tachycardia
and, 264, 265
posture and, 313
vaso-vagal, 314
Syphilis
complete heart block in, 296
Syringomyelia
orthostatic hypotension and, 318

T

T-waves, lowering of, 166
T-waves, peaked, 158
Tabes dorsalis, 318
Tamponade
acute pericarditis and, 103
anticoagulant therapy and, 77
dissecting aneurysm of aorta and,
90, 91
Tension pneumothorax, 96
Tent-shaped T-wave
potassium intoxication and, 158
Tetralogy of Fallot
syncope in, 325
Therapeutic–toxic ratio
digitalis and, 173
Thomas collar
nerve root pain and, 99
Thoracentesis
congestive heart failure and, 136
digitalis intoxication and, 175
Thoracotomy
cardiac resuscitation and, 338–345
venous air embolism and, 359
Thorazine, 334
Thrombectomy
acute pulmonary embolism and, 125
Thrombolytic agents
arterial and venous thromboses and,
78
Thrombophlebitis
elastic stockings and, 127
pulmonary embolism and, 124–128
Thrombosis
thrombolytic agents for, 78
Thyroidectomy incision
acute mediastinal emphysema
treated by, 96
Thyrotoxic heart disease
atrial fibrillation in, 257
digitalis requirement in, 256

paroxysmal atrial tachycardia and, 193
paroxysmal ventricular tachycardia in, 264
"refractory" congestive failure and, 135
Thyrotoxicosis
angina pectoris and, 57
Tietze's syndrome, 104, 105
Tight collar
carotid sinus sensitivity and, 317
Tinnitis, 228, 284
Tissue necrosis
nor-epinephrine and, 43
Tourniquets
(see venous tourniquets)
Tracheal suction
syncope during, 322
Tranquilizing agents, 318, 334
Transaminase, serum
pulmonary infarction and, 120
Transfusion
Dicumarol toxicity and, 71
packed red cells and, 29
shock and, 40
of incompatible blood
potassium intoxication from, 156
Transperitoneal dialysis
potassium intoxication treated with, 163
Trendelenburg operation
acute pulmonary embolism and, 125
Trendelenburg position
shock and, 40
Tromexan
(see ethyl biscoumacetate)
Tubular necrosis, acute
potassium intoxication in, 156
Tussive syncope, 321

U

U-waves, prominent, 166
Ulceration of esophagus
hiatus hernia and, 107
Uremia, 156
Urine, fat in
fat embolism and, 360
Uterine bleeding
anticoagulant therapy and, 77

V

Valsalva maneuver, 204, 321, 322

Varicose veins, 320
Vasoconstriction, 40, 42
Vaso-pressor amines
digitalis–potentiating action of, 46
orthostatic hypotension and, 319
paroxysmal atrial tachycardia and, 207
paroxysmal ventricular tachycardia treated with, 279, 285
shock and, 40–46
Vaso-vagal syncope, 314
Vasoxyl (see methoxamine)
Vena cava, superior, dilatation of
acute cor pulmonale and, 121
Venous air embolism
left lateral decubitus, 359
Venous thrombosis
thrombolytic agents for, 78
Venous tourniquet
acute left ventricular failure and, 17, 23–25
Ventricular capture
atrioventricular dissociation and, 185
paroxysmal ventricular tachycardia and, 271
Ventricular fibrillation
complete heart block and, 296
digitalis intoxication and, 185
external defibrillator for, 305, 339, 345, 346, 347
manual systole for, 339, 345, 346
potassium for, 346
potassium intoxication and, 160
Ventricular flutter
complete heart block and, 292
potassium intoxication and, 160, 285
Ventricular premature beats
aberrant ventricular conduction and, 180
digitalis intoxication and, 179
quinidine and, 220
Ventricular standstill
blow to chest for, 305
complete heart block and, 292
intracranial surgery and, 334
calcium chloride and, 339
epinephrine and, 339
external pacemaker and, 305, 346
"internal" pacemaker and, 339
needle stimulation of heart for, 305

paroxysmal atrial tachycardia followed by, 207
post-tachycardial, 305
potassium intoxication and, 160
Ventricular tachycardia
(see paroxysmal ventricular tachycardia)
Vertebrae, percussion of
nerve root pain and, 98
Vertebral fracture
chest pain and, 97
"Vicious cycle"
shock and, 40
Viral pericarditis
(see acute pericarditis)
Vital capacity of lungs
"arm chair" treatment and, 137
Vitamin K_1 oxide, 69, 71

Vomiting, 22, 165, 176, 284

W

"Water intoxication," 146
Wolff-Parkinson-White syndrome
paroxysmal atrial tachycardia and, 193
Wyamine
(see mephentermine)
Warfarin sodium
(see coumadin sodium)

X

X-ray
(see Roentgen-ray)

Y

Yellow vision, 177, 178